MCQ Tutor in Radiology FRCR Part I

MCQ Tutor in Radiology FRCR Part I

Andrea L. Brown MRCP (UK) FRCR
Senior Registrar in Radiology, Northwick Park Hospital, London

Lesley A. Apthorp MA, MRCP (UK) FRCR
Senior Registrar in Radiology, Guy's and St Thomas' Hospitals, London
Previously Registrar in Radiology, Northwick Park Hsopital, London

Uday S. Bhonsle MSc, MIPSM
Consultant Physicist, Northwick Park Hospital, London

Edited by
Gerald de Lacey MA, FRCR
Consultant Radiologist, Northwick Park Hospital, London

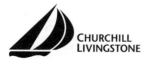

CHURCHILL
LIVINGSTONE

NEW YORK EDINBURGH LONDON MADRID MELBOURNE SAN FRANCISCO
TOKYO 1996

CHURCHILL LIVINGSTONE
Medical Division of Pearson Professional Limited

Distributed in the United States of America by Churchill
Livingstone Inc., 650 Avenue of the Americas, New
York, N.Y. 10011, and by associated companies,
branches and representatives throughout the world.

First edition 1996

ISBN 0 443 05464 9

British Library of Cataloguing in Publication Data
A catalogue record for this book is available from the
British Library.

Library of Congress Cataloging in Publication Data
A catalog record for this book is available from the
Library of Congress.

Medical knowledge is constantly changing. As new information becomes
available, changes in treatment, procedures, equipment and the use of drugs
become necessary. The authors and the publishers have, as far as it is
possible, taken care to ensure that the information given in this text is accurate
and up to date. However, readers are strongly advised to confirm that the
information, especially with regard to drug usage, complies with current
legislation and standards of practice.

The
publisher's
policy is to use
**paper manufactured
from sustainable forests**

Produced by Longman Singapore Publishers (Pte) Ltd.
Printed in Singapore

Contents

Foreword

It is a pleasure to write a foreword to this excellent book of Multiple Choice Questions (MCQs). Now that most examinations in radiology are entirely based on MCQs, there is a need for a large bank for learning and self testing. And, as stated in the introduction, practice will indicate where improvements in technique and knowledge are required.

The authors have done a very good job in making the questions as unambiguous as possible and making them relevant to the practice of modern radiology. I suspect that the book has largely arisen through the endeavours of the two young radiologist first authors who have recently passed the Part I FRCR examination. They have wisely solicited the help of a physicist who has contributed some very up-to-date physics questions and that of a senior radiologist with considerable examining experience who has kept them on the straight and narrow. This team has provided 300 first class questions. As a previous examiner, I know just how hard it is to compose realistic questions of the right degree of difficulty.

There is a lot of new material here with many of the physics questions involving MRI, PET and the like. It is of course difficult to make the anatomy questions seem 'trendy', but even here there are some intriguing new concepts.

It is pleasing that the answers are provided on the opposite page which makes life so much easier than having to look them up at the end. There are also useful comments admixed with the answers which make the book a really worthwhile educational exercise. I have certainly learnt a lot from it.

I have no doubt that the book will be well received in all countries. The questions are those that all radiologists should be able to answer. Thus it should appeal to specialist registrars and qualified radiologists alike. Of course with increasing pressure on specialist registrars to attain their goals in each year of training, first year trainees will be the chief purchasers. And it will sell well. But more than mere sales, I think that the material within this volume will become a standard text for trainees and trainers. And thus the authors have achieved a lot. They should be thanked and congratulated for their efforts. I wish them, the publication team and the book well.

Adrian K Dixon MD FRCR FRCP
Professor of Radiology
University of Cambridge

Introduction

In June 1993 a revised syllabus was introduced for the FRCR part I examination of the Royal College of Radiologists. There were three major changes: the written part of the examination was limited to multiple choice questions (MCQs); the amount of physics was reduced so as to achieve the objectives that candidates should have a sound understanding of the processes which occurred once the X-rays had left the X-ray tube and that there would be considerably less emphasis on what actually happened inside the tube and generator; and finally, some imaging modalities (CT and MRI) were given an increased prominence.

It is intended that this book should be used during the early stages of organised study and so assist with the written part of the FRCR part I examination taking into account the new syllabus (page 208).

There are a total of 300 MCQs arranged into three separate sections reflecting the three main sections (anatomy, techniques and physics) of the FRCR part I examination.

ACKNOWLEDGEMENTS

The authors are greatly indebted to Dr P.P. Dendy, Chief Physicist, Medical Physics Department, Addenbrookes Hospital, Cambridge and Mr G. Manson, Principal Physicist, Medical Physics Department, Cork University Hospital, Ireland. Their helpful comments and suggestions on the physics section of this book have been invaluable. The Royal College of Radiologists has kindly given permission to the authors to include the present FRCR I syllabus in this book.

The FRCR part I examination

Candidates are permitted to sit the examination after one academic year's preparation in a training post which has been approved by the Royal College of Radiologists. Examinations are held in June and September each year. The examination has three components:

I. One multiple choice question (MCQ) paper (2 hours)

- A total of 60 questions distributed equally between anatomy, techniques, and physics (i.e. 20 questions in each area).

- Each question has a stem followed by five independent items or statements. Each statement is either true or false.

- There is no restriction on the number of true or false items in a question. It is possible for all five components to be true or all five to be false.

- The scoring system is as follows:
  for each item correctly indicated as true or false   +1
  for each item incorrectly indicated   −1
  for each item indicated "don't know"   0

- MCQ syntax:
  - *The majority* means more than 50%
  - The approved name of a drug is always utilised; sometimes the proprietary name will be added in brackets.

II. One film viewing session (1 hour)

- This is designed to test the candidate's knowledge of radiological anatomy, radiographic techniques and understanding of film faults. Films are displayed on viewing boxes and each candidate is required to answer four questions on each radiograph. There are a total of 20 radiographs and thus a total of 80 questions.

- All the questions are attached to the radiograph and the candidate records his/her answers in a book.

- An invigilator and several examiners are present. Candidates are not questioned by the examiners who are present during this part of the examination.

III. Two oral examinations (20 minutes each)

● All candidates proceed to the oral examinations.

● Each candidate is examined by two pairs of examiners. One pair consists of a physicist and a clinical radiologist who examine in physics. The second pair consists of two clinical radiologists who examine in anatomy and techniques.

How to use this book

- The MCQs are grouped together under three sections:
  - anatomy
  - techniques
  - physics.

- Each section comprises 100 questions.

- Each question has a stem, followed by five independent statements.

- The correct answers are indicated on the right-hand page opposite each question. In many instances the answers include a short explanation.

- A glossary of abbreviations is provided on page xiv.

- A bibliography containing a list of the texts which have been used to formulate the MCQ questions is included on page 206.

- The FRCR part I syllabus is included on pages 208–213.

- An index of all the subjects which have been included in the MCQs is listed alphabetically on pages 215–227.

Note: some explanations given within the physics MCQ answers may be an approximation for the purposes of illustration of a principle.

Answering multiple choice questions

The majority of candidates will have had experience of sitting multiple choice question (MCQ) papers at undergraduate and postgraduate level. Therefore **the most important advice is for a candidate not to change his/her technique when it has been successful in the past.**

Three practical tips:

1. **Attempt enough questions.** Answer at least 240 items out of the total of 300 (60×5) items in order to score enough positive marks to pass the MCQ examination.

   The principle behind this advice is as follows. Assuming that a candidate has an error rate of 10%, then:

   - the candidate should pass with a clear margin if 240 questions are attempted as the net positive score will be 192 or 64% (i.e. 216 correct answers less 24 incorrect answers).
   - a marginal pass or fail would be likely when the candidate attempts only 200 questions, as the net positive score would be 160 or 53% (i.e. 180 correct answers less 20 incorrect answers).
   - the candidate is likely to fail if only 160 questions are answered as the net positive score would be 128 or 43% (i.e. 144 correct answers less 16 incorrect answers).

   Obviously the assumed error rate of 10% (for all answers which have confidently been assumed to be correct) will vary between different individuals. A candidate should therefore assess his or her own personal error rate by doing test examination papers and comparing the number of statements incorrectly answered with the total number of questions attempted. Based on this estimated average error rate, an approximation of the minimum number of items which should be answered to achieve a clear pass can be determined by using the previous example as a guide.

2. **Do not guess randomly.** On the other hand it is recognised that intelligent guesses often give a net positive rather than a net negative score. A candidate should assess his or her own personal success rate on several test MCQ papers by comparing scores before and after additional intelligent responses. The results

should allow each candidate to develop the most profitable answering style.

3. **Practice makes perfect**. Practice on test MCQ papers will indicate where improvements in technique and knowledge are required.

FURTHER READING

1. Anderson J. *The Multiple Choice Question in Medicine*, 2nd edn. London: Pitman, 1982.
2. Holden NL. Multiple-choice questions : a guide to success. *Br J Hosp Med* 1993; **50** (**9**): 557–559.
3. Robinson PJ. Strategic marking in MCQ papers (letter). *Br J Radiol* 1981; **54**: 538–539.

Glossary

Throughout the text the following abbreviations have been used:

ADC	Analogue–digital converter
AP	Anteroposterior
ARSAC	Administration of Radioactive Substances Advisory Committee
^{11}C	Carbon-11
^{12}C	Carbon-12
^{13}C	Carbon-13
^{14}C	Carbon-14
^{60}Co	Cobalt-60
COR	Centre of rotation
CT	Computed tomography
DMSA	Dimercaptosuccinic acid
DSA	Digital subtraction angiography
DTPA	Diethylene triamine pentaacetic acid
ECG	Electrocardiograph
EDE	Effective dose equivalent
ERCP	Endoscopic retrograde cholangiopancreatography
^{18}F	Fluorine-18
FID	Free induction decay
FOV	Field of view
^{67}Ga	Gallium-67
^{1}H	Hydrogen-1
(H)IDA	(Hepatic) iminodiacetic acid
HMPAO	Hexamethyl propylene amine oxime
HOCM	High-osmolar contrast medium
HSG	Hysterosalpingography
HVT	Half value thickness
IADSA	Intra-arterial digital subtraction angiography
ICRP	International Commission on Radiological Protection
IRR	Ionising Radiation(s) Regulations
IV	Intravenous
IVDSA	Intravenous digital subtraction angiography
IVU	Intravenous urogram
^{40}K	Potassium-40
LAO	Left anterior oblique

LET	Linear energy transfer
LOCM	Low-osmolar contrast medium
LPO	Left posterior oblique
LSF	Line spread function
MAG	Benzoylmercaptoacetyltriglycerine
MDP	Methylene diphosphonate
MIBG	M-iodobenzylguanidine
MIBI	Methoxy isobutyl isonitrile
MRA	Magnetic resonance angiography
MR(I)	Magnetic resonance (imaging)
MTF	Modulation transfer function
^{13}N	Nitrogen-13
^{14}N	Nitrogen-14
^{15}N	Nitrogen-15
NMV	Net magnetisation vector
^{15}O	Oxygen-15
OF	Occipitofrontal
OM	Occipitomental
^{31}P	Phosphorus-31
PA	Posteroanterior
PET	Positron emission tomography
POPUMET	Protection of Persons Undergoing Medical Examinations or Treatment (The Ionising Radiation Regulations. Statutory Instrument No. 778)
PMT	Photomultiplier tube
PRF	Pulse repetition frequency
PTC	Percutaneous transhepatic cholangiography
RAO	Right anterior oblique
^{222}Rn	Radon-222
RBE	Relative biological effectiveness
RF	Radiofrequency
RPO	Right posterior oblique
SE	Spin echo
SPECT	Single photon emission computed tomography
STIR	Short T1-Inversion Recovery
^{99m}Tc	Technetium-99m
TE	Echo time
^{201}Tl	Thallium-201
TOF	Time of flight
TR	Repetition time
TV	Television
^{127}Xe	Xenon-127
^{133}Xe	Xenon-133

1 Anatomy

1 **The following have usually begun to ossify at birth:**
   A the patella.
   B the lower femoral epiphysis.
   C the navicular.
   D the capitulum.
   E the pisiform.

2 **In the normal wrist:**
   A the scaphoid and the lunate articulate with the distal radius.
   B the scaphoid and the lunate articulate with the head of the capitate.
   C the pisiform articulates with the posterior surface of the triquetrum.
   D the trapezium and trapezoid articulate with the scaphoid.
   E the proximal part of the triquetrum articulates with the ulna.

3 **In the wrist:**
   A the triquetrum lies in the distal carpal row.
   B the radiocarpal joint communicates with the midcarpal joint.
   C the pisiform is the only carpal bone to give attachment to both the flexor and extensor retinaculae.
   D the scaphoid is the most anterior carpal bone on a true lateral radiograph.
   E the capitate is usually ossified at birth.

1 A **False**   Appears at about 5 years of age.
   B **True**   Appears at about 37 weeks gestation.
   C **False**   Usually the last of the tarsal bones to ossify. The
                   ossification centre for the navicular appears at about
                   4 years of age.
   D **False**   Appears at about 1 year and is the first ossification
                   centre to be seen at the elbow. It is usually (but not
                   always) followed by the radial head, internal
                   epicondyle, trochlea, olecranon and external
                   epicondyle.
   E **False**   Appears at about 11 years of age and is the last
                   carpal bone to ossify.

2 A **True**
   B **True**
   C **False**   The pisiform articulates with the anterior surface of
                   the triquetrum.
   D **True**
   E **False**   The proximal part of the triquetrum articulates with
                   the triangular articular disc of the wrist joint.

3 A **False**   The proximal carpal row comprises the scaphoid, the
                   lunate, the triquetrum and the pisiform. The distal
                   row comprises the trapezium, the trapezoid, the
                   capitate and the hamate.
   B **False**   The radiocarpal joint does not communicate with the
                   midcarpal joint in the normal wrist. The midcarpal
                   joint communicates with the carpometacarpal joint.
   C **True**   The flexor retinaculum attaches to the scaphoid
                   tubercle and ridge of the trapezium laterally, and the
                   pisiform and hook of the hamate medially. The
                   extensor retinaculum attaches to the radius, pisiform
                   and triquetral bones.
   D **False**   The pisiform is the most anterior carpal bone.
   E **False**   The capitate usually ossifies at about 4 months.

4 In the normal shoulder:
  A the joint capsule is lax inferiorly.
  B the normal acromiohumeral distance is greater than 7 mm.
  C the glenohumeral joint normally communicates with the
       subacromial bursa.
  D the normal glenohumeral joint space has a maximum width of
       6 mm.
  E the rotator cuff muscles all insert into the lesser tuberosity of
       the humerus.

5 In the normal shoulder joint:
  A the long tendon of biceps is extracapsular.
  B the capsule is attached to the articular margin of the humeral
       head except at the inferior margin.
  C the subacromial bursa extends inwards under the acromion
       when the arm is abducted.
  D the "rotator cuff" comprises the fused tendons of
       subscapularis, supraspinatus, infraspinatus and teres major.
  E the articular surface of the humeral head is four times the area
       of the glenoid.

6 Regarding the arterial supply to the upper limb:
  A the deep palmar arch is formed from the continuation of the
       radial artery.
  B the axillary artery lies lateral to the axillary vein.
  C the axillary artery becomes the brachial artery at the lower
       border of teres minor.
  D the axillary artery is divided into three parts by the pectoralis
       minor muscle.
  E the axillary artery commences at the medial border of the first
       rib.

4 A True   The joint capsule passes round the circumference of the glenoid fossa extending proximally to include the root of the coracoid process and distally onto the anatomical neck of the humerus. It is strong, but is lax inferiorly and so allows a wide range of movement.

   B True   A distance less than 5 mm suggests a rotator cuff tear.

   C False   The subacromical bursa does not normally communicate with the glenohumeral joint. However, the subscapular bursa does communicate with the synovial membrane of the glenohumeral joint.

   D True   If greater than 6 mm it is suggestive of a posterior dislocation.

   E False   Supraspinatus, infraspinatus and teres minor insert into the greater tuberosity of the humerus. Subscapularis is inserted into the lesser tuberosity.

---

5 A False   It is intracapsular.

   B True   Inferiorly, the capsule is attached to the neck of the humerus below the articular margin.

   C True   However, the subacromial bursa extends beyond the lateral border of the acromion with the arm adducted.

   D False   It comprises the fused tendons of subscapularis, supraspinatus, infraspinatus and teres minor.

   E True

---

6 A True   The deep palmar arch is formed from the terminal branch of the radial artery anastomosing with the deep branch of the ulnar artery. The superficial arch is formed from the continuation of the ulnar artery.

   B True

   C False   The axillary artery becomes the brachial artery at the lower border of teres major.

   D True   The first part is above pectoralis minor and has one branch; the second part is behind pectoralis minor and has two branches; the third part is below pectoralis minor and has three branches.

   E False   The axillary artery commences at the lateral border of the first rib.

7   In the knee:

A   the fabella lies in the lateral head of the gastrocnemius muscle in about 80% of the population.

B   the superomedial aspect of the patella may ossify independently and remain discrete.

C   the posterior cruciate ligament is attached to the anterior intercondylar area of the tibia.

D   the lateral collateral ligament is attached to the lateral meniscus.

E   the lateral articular surface of the patella is larger than the medial articular surface.

8   The following are true:

A   the suprapatellar bursa communicates with the knee joint.

B   the gastrocnemius bursa may communicate with the medial condylar cavity of the knee joint.

C   the medial meniscus of the knee joint is larger than the lateral meniscus.

D   the collateral ligaments of the knee joint are extracapsular.

E   the popliteus tendon is intracapsular.

9   The patella:

A   is a sesamoid bone.

B   is bipartite in 2% of cases.

C   commonly has an irregular anterior margin.

D   has two paired facets on its posterior surface.

E   forms an attachment for the capsule of the knee joint.

7 A False The fabella, a sesamoid bone, lies in the lateral head of the gastrocnemius muscle in about 22% of the population.

B False The superolateral aspect of the patella occasionally ossifies independently and remains discrete. This is referred to as a bipartite patella.

C False The posterior cruciate ligament is attached to the posterior intercondylar area and passes anteriorly, medially and superiorly to the lateral aspect of the medial femoral condyle.

D False The lateral collateral ligament is separate from the lateral meniscus. It is attached superiorly to the lateral epicondyle of the femur and inferiorly to the head of the fibula. However, the deep part of the medial collateral ligament is attached to the medial meniscus.

E True

8 A True
B True In about 43% of individuals.
C True The lateral meniscus is more rounded than the medial which is more crescentic in shape.
D True On the other hand the anterior and posterior cruciate ligaments of the knee joint are intracapsular, but extrasynovial.
E True The popliteus tendon separates the lateral meniscus, to which it is attached, from the lateral collateral ligament of the knee joint.

9 A True A sesamoid is a fibrous, cartilaginous or bony nodule within a tendon. The only constant examples are the patella, which is the largest, and one in each of the two tendons of flexor pollicis brevis in the hand, and flexor hallucis brevis in the foot.

B True A bipartite patella occurs much more commonly in males than females. When present, this normal variant occurs bilaterally in 43% of cases.

C True
D False On the posterior surface of the patella, there are three paired facets for articulation with the patellar surface of the femur. There is also a medial facet for articulation, in full flexion, with the medial margin of the intercondylar notch of the femur.

E True

10   In the normal hip:

   A the ischiofemoral ligament is the strongest of the three ligaments.

   B the joint capsule attaches to the intertrochanteric crest posteriorly.

   C the artery of the ligamentum teres originates from the obturator artery.

   D the angle of inclination of the femoral neck is normally about 127° in adults.

   E the ossification centre for the femoral head is visible at birth.

11   The femoral artery:

   A is a continuation of the external iliac artery beyond the inguinal ligament.

   B becomes the popliteal artery after piercing adductor magnus.

   C lies anterior to the femoral vein in the adductor canal.

   D supplies branches to the skin of the anterior abdominal wall.

   E gives rise to the profunda femoris artery in the femoral triangle.

12   Regarding the veins of the lower limb:

   A the long saphenous vein lies anterior to the medial malleolus.

   B the long saphenous vein contains less than five valves.

   C the short saphenous vein lies with the sural nerve anterior to the lateral malleolus.

   D there is no communication between the short and long saphenous veins.

   E the long saphenous vein drains into the popliteal vein.

10 A False   The iliofemoral ligament (Y-shaped ligament of Bigelow) is the strongest ligament around the hip. The ischiofemoral ligament is the weakest ligament. The pubofemoral ligament is the third ligament around the hip.

    B False   Posteriorly the joint capsule does not extend as far as the intertrochanteric crest. It is attached halfway along the femoral neck. Anteriorly the joint capsule is attached to the intertrochanteric line.

    C True

    D True   In neonates, the angle of inclination is normally 160°. The angle of anteversion is 50° at birth and 8° in adults.

    E False   It appears during the first year of life.

---

11 A True

    B True

    C True   In the femoral sheath, the femoral artery lies lateral to the femoral vein. It changes position relative to the femoral vein as it passes from the femoral sheath downwards into the adductor canal.

    D True   The femoral artery gives off superficial branches which supply the anterior abdominal wall and skin of the external genitalia.

    E True

---

12 A True

    B False   The long saphenous vein contains at least 10 valves.

    C False   The short saphenous vein lies with the sural nerve posterior to the lateral malleolus.

    D False   There are several channels of communication between the short and long saphenous veins.

    E False   The long saphenous vein drains into the femoral vein. The short saphenous vein drains into the popliteal vein.

13   The clavicle:

A   ossifies in membrane.

B   has a secondary ossification centre at its lateral end which appears at 18 years and fuses at 25 years.

C   forms a secondary cartilaginous joint with the sternum.

D   has a rhomboid fossa in approximately 0.5% of the population.

E   may exhibit a conoid tubercle for attachment of the costoclavicular ligament.

14   Regarding the ribs:

A   the first costal cartilage to ossify is most commonly that of the first rib.

B   all the ribs have two facets for the costovertebral joints.

C   the tubercle of a typical rib forms a synovial joint with the transverse process of its own vertebra.

D   cervical ribs occur in approximately 1.5% of people.

E   each rib forms a secondary cartilaginous joint with its costal cartilage.

15   Regarding the major airways:

A   the trachea bifurcates at the level of T5.

B   the normal subcarinal angle is approximately 90°.

C   the right main bronchus is both more vertical and longer than the left.

D   the trachea is reinforced by 15–20 incomplete rings of hyaline cartilage.

E   on a lateral chest radiograph, the right upper lobe bronchus is visualised end on above the left main stem bronchus.

13 A True   It has no medullary cavity.
    B False   The secondary ossification centre is at the modial
                end of the clavicle.
    C False   The sternoclavicular joint is a synovial joint with an
                intra-articular fibrocartilaginous disc dividing the joint
                in two. The manubriosternal joint is a secondary
                cartilaginous joint.
    D True   A rhomboid fossa occurs in 0.6% of normal clavicles.
                33% of these are bilateral.
    E False   The conoid tubercle is for attachment of the conoid
                part of the coracoclavicular ligament. The rhomboid
                fossa is the site of attachment for the costoclavicular
                ligament.

14 A True   Ossification of the first costal cartilage often starts in
                the second or third decade. The costal cartilages of
                the lowest ribs ossify next and the process
                progresses upwards.
    B False   A typical rib has two facets. The lower facet forms a
                synovial joint with the upper costal facet of its own
                vertebra and the upper facet with the lower costal
                facet of the vertebra above. However, the first rib has
                only one costovertebral facet and articulates with T1
                vertebra only.
    C True   The tubercle of a typical rib has two facets. The
                medial facet forms a synovial joint with the
                transverse process of its own vertebra. The lateral
                facet is non-articular and gives attachment to the
                lateral costotransverse ligament.
    D True   They are usually bilateral but asymmetric in size.
    E False   They are primary cartilaginous joints. A primary
                cartilaginous joint is where bone and hyaline
                cartilage meet; a secondary cartilaginous joint
                (symphysis) is a union between bones whose
                articular surfaces are covered with a thin lamina of
                hyaline cartilage.

15 A True   It bifurcates at the lower level of T5.
    B False   The normal subcarinal angle is 60° ± 10° standard
                deviation.
    C False   The right main bronchus is more vertical than the
                left, but shorter. The right main bronchus measures
                2.5 cm in length and the left measures 5 cm.
    D True
    E True

16   The trachea is an immediate relation of:
 A   the left vagus nerve.
 B   the oesophagus.
 C   the isthmus of the thyroid gland.
 D   the thoracic duct.
 E   the left brachiocephalic vein.

17   Regarding the fissures of the lung:
 A   all the accessory fissures comprise two layers of visceral pleura.
 B   the minor fissure runs horizontally on the right at the level of fourth costal cartilage.
 C   the azygos fissure occurs in about 5% of normal individuals.
 D   on the lateral chest radiograph the left oblique fissure is usually more vertical than the right.
 E   the inferior accessory fissure separates the lateral basal segment of the right lower lobe from the rest of the lobe.

18   At the pulmonary hilum:
 A   the density seen on a plain chest radiograph is mainly due to lymph nodes and bronchi.
 B   the transverse diameter of the basal pulmonary artery is approximately 15 mm in an adult female.
 C   the left pulmonary artery passes anterior to the left main bronchus throughout its course.
 D   the hilar point is where the basal pulmonary artery crosses the upper lobe vein.
 E   the right hilum is higher than the left in about 5% of people.

16 A False The right vagus nerve is in contact with the trachea. The left is held away from the trachea by the great vessels and aortic arch.

B True The oesophagus is a direct posterior relation of the trachea.

C True The isthmus of the thyroid gland is an anterior relation of the trachea.

D False The thoracic duct passes from right to left, posterior to the oesophagus, at the level of T5.

E False

---

17 A False The azygos has four layers. All the others have two layers of visceral pleura.

B True

C False It occurs in about 1% of normal individuals. It is visualised on 0.1% of chest radiographs.

D True The left oblique fissure therefore meets the diaphragm more posteriorly than the right.

E False The inferior accessory fissure separates the medial basal segment of the lower lobe from the rest of the lobe. It occurs in about 25% of individuals, making it the most common accessory fissure.

---

18 A False The density of the normal hilum is mainly due to blood vessels.

B True It measures approximately 16 mm in men.

C False The left pulmonary artery initially lies anterior to the bronchus, then arches over the left main bronchus to lie posterior to it. The right pulmonary artery lies anterior to the right main bronchus.

D True The hilar angle is formed by the intersection of the basal pulmonary artery and the upper lobe vein and is normally about 120°.

E False The right hilum is higher than the left in about 0.05% of people. The hila are at the same level in about 3% of cases. In the remaining 97% of cases the left hilum is higher than the right.

19 On a normal PA chest radiograph:

A the left paraspinal line is wider than the right.
B the maximum width of the right paratracheal line is 3 mm.
C the azygos vein should not have a diameter greater than 5 mm.
D the posterior junction line extends above the suprasternal notch and comprises four layers of pleura.
E the aortic nipple is formed by the left superior intercostal vein arching around the aortic arch.

20 In the lung:

A the left upper lobe is divided into three segments.
B the bronchial arteries all arise directly from the aorta.
C the lingula is divided into medial and lateral segments.
D an acinus comprises three to five terminal bronchioles.
E the veins are usually anterior to the arteries.

21 Regarding the pulmonary vasculature:

A the lower zone veins are more vertical than their corresponding arteries.
B the normal mean pulmonary arterial pressure is approximately 15 mmHg.
C the truncus anterior arises from the right pulmonary artery at the hilum.
D the pulmonary trunk is a posterior relation of the left atrium.
E in the upper lobes the veins usually lie lateral to the arteries.

22 At the level of the lower border of T4:

A the left phrenic nerve lies adjacent to the trachea.
B the thoracic duct lies anterior to the oesophagus.
C the azygos vein joins the superior vena cava.
D the second costal cartilage meets the manubrio-sternal joint.
E the ligamentum arteriosum is situated.

19 A True   The maximum diameter of the right paraspinal line is 2 mm. The maximum width of the left paraspinal line is 1 cm.

B True

C False   The azygos vein has a maximum diameter of 1 cm.

D True   Whereas the anterior junction line ends below the suprasternal notch.

E True

---

20 A False   The left upper lobe comprises apicoposterior and anterior segments and the lingula comprises superior and inferior segments.

B False   There are usually three bronchial arteries, two on the left arising directly from the aorta, and one on the right arising from the third right posterior intercostal artery.

C False   The lingula is divided into superior and inferior segments. The right middle lobe is divided into medial and lateral segments.

D False   A secondary lobule comprises three to five terminal bronchioles. An acinus is all the lung parenchyma distal to one terminal bronchiole.

E True

---

21 A False   Lower zone veins tend to be more horizontal than the arteries. In the upper zones, the veins are more vertical than the arteries.

B True   Mean pulmonary venous pressure is approximately 3 mmHg.

C False   The truncus anterior arises proximal to the hilum and passes to supply the right upper lobe.

D False   The pulmonary trunk is anterior to the left atrium.

E True

---

22 A False   It is separated from the trachea by the arch of the aorta.

B False   The thoracic duct crosses from right to left as it ascends posterior to the oesophagus at the level of T4/T5.

C True

D True   The manubrio-sternal angle lies at the level of T4.

E True   This is the remnant of the ductus arteriosus, which connects the left pulmonary artery to the aorta in fetal life. It lies in the aortopulmonary window.

23   The superior vena cava:

   A   is formed at the level of T7.
   B   has two valves.
   C   has only one tributary.
   D   is an immediate relation of the right phrenic nerve.
   E   may be left sided.

24   Regarding the azygos venous system:

   A   embryologically the azygos vein develops from the right
        posterior cardinal vein.
   B   the azygos vein is formed from the union of the ascending
        lumbar and right subcostal veins.
   C   it commences at the level of L5.
   D   the hemiazygos vein crosses from left to right at the level of
        T8 to join the azygos vein.
   E   the accessory hemiazygos vein receives bronchial veins from
        the left lung.

25   The thoracic duct:

   A   commences as a continuation of the cisterna chyli at the level
        of L4.
   B   passes through the central tendon of the diaphragm at the
        level of T12.
   C   has no valves.
   D   drains the lymph from the whole thorax.
   E   crosses the posterior mediastinum from right to left and is
        then anterior to the oesophagus at the level of T5.

26   Regarding lymphatic drainage:

   A   the right lymphatic duct drains into the right brachiocephalic
        vein.
   B   the thoracic duct has a diameter of 10–12 mm.
   C   the thoracic duct is approximately 45 cm long.
   D   the thoracic duct drains into the azygos vein.
   E   the thoracic duct lies between the azygos vein and the
        descending aorta in the lower mediastinum.

23 A **False**   It commences behind the manubrium (T3/4) and
                   enters the right atrium.
    B **False**   It has no valves.
    C **True**   The azygos vein drains into it posteriorly at T4.
    D **True**
    E **True**   In 0.3% of people.

24 A **True**
    B **True**
    C **False**   It commences in front of and slightly to the right of
                   L2, and ascends to the right of the vertebral column.
    D **True**   It passes posterior to the oesophagus, and receives
                   the lower eight posterior intercostal veins.
    E **True**   It also receives some veins from the middle third of
                   the oesophagus.

25 A **False**   It commences at L1.
    B **False**   It passes between the overlapping right and left
                   crural fibres, behind the median arcuate ligament at
                   the level of T12.
    C **False**   There are many valves, the last of which is
                   approximately 5 cm proximal to the venous junction.
    D **False**   It drains the whole body below the diaphragm and
                   the left half above it. The right side of the thorax,
                   head and neck drain into the right lymphatic duct.
    E **False**   It crosses the posterior mediastinum posterior to the
                   oesophagus.

26 A **True**   It drains the right side of the thorax, right arm, head
                   and neck.
    B **False**   The diameter of the thoracic duct is 1–7 mm.
    C **True**   The cisterna chyli is 6 cm long.
    D **False**   The thoracic duct enters the point of confluence of
                   the left internal jugular and subclavian veins at the
                   level of C7.
    E **True**   The azygos vein lies to the right of the thoracic duct
                   and the descending aorta to its left.

27 The thymus:
A   is usually situated in the anterior mediastinum.
B   is predominantly composed of fatty tissue in young children.
C   reaches its maximum weight at 2 years.
D   consists of two lobes, the right is usually larger than the left.
E   receives its blood supply from the inferior thyroid and internal thoracic arteries.

28   The following are situated in the aortopulmonary window:
A   the ductus node.
B   the left recurrent laryngeal nerve.
C   the left bronchial artery.
D   the left vagus nerve.
E   the ligamentum arteriosum.

29 The oesophagus:
A   commences at the cricopharyngeus muscle at C4.
B   pierces the diaphragm with the right phrenic nerve.
C   has striated muscle in the wall of its upper third, and smooth muscle in the wall more distally.
D   is retroperitoneal in its intra-abdominal portion.
E   receives part of its blood supply from the thyrocervical trunk.

30   The following impress on the oesophagus as follows:
A   The lower fibres of the inferior constrictor muscle of the pharynx cause a posterior impression.
B   The post-cricoid venous plexus causes a posterior impression.
C   The aortic knuckle at the level of T6.
D   The left main bronchus as it passes posterior to the oesophagus.
E   An aberrant right subclavian artery causes an anterior impression.

27 A **True**   It lies anterior to the great vessels and trachea.
    B **False**   It comprises lymphoid and epithelial cells in childhood, which are replaced by fatty tissue in adult life.
    C **False**   It weighs 10–15 g at birth, grows for 2 years and then stops growing until 7 years when it has a second growth spurt, reaching a maximum weight of 30–40 g at 11 years.
    D **True**
    E **True**

28 A **True**
    B **True**
    C **True**   All these are situated in the aortopulmonary window, along with fat.
    D **True**
    E **True**

29 A **False**   It commences at the cricopharyngeus muscle at C6.
    B **False**   It passes through the diaphragm at the level of T10 accompanied by branches of the left gastric artery and both vagus nerves (left anteriorly, right posteriorly).
    C **True**   This probably accounts for the fact that normal physiological events occur more quickly in the upper oesophagus.
    D **True**   The distal 3 cm is retroperitoneal.
    E **True**   The upper oesophagus is supplied by the inferior thyroid artery from the thyrocervical trunk; the middle portion by oesophageal branches of the aorta; and the lower portion by branches of the left gastric artery.

30 A **True**   This is the cricopharyngeus muscle.
    B **False**   This venous plexus commonly causes anterior impressions at C6.
    C **False**   The aortic knuckle may cause a left sided impression at T4.
    D **False**   The left main bronchus indents the oesophagus as it passes in front of it.
    E **False**   An aberrant right subclavian artery causes a posterior impression.

31 In the larynx:

A the corniculate cartilages commonly ossify.
B each pyriform fossa lies between the aryepiglottic membrane medially, and the lamina of the thyroid cartilage laterally.
C the vestibule separates the true and false vocal cords.
D the triticeal cartilage lies in the thyrohyoid membrane.
E the valleculae are paired depressions at the base of the tongue situated between the tongue and the epiglottis.

32 In the region of the larynx:

A the hyoid bone is situated at the level of C3.
B the thyroid cartilage is situated at the level of C6.
C the cricoarytenoid articulations are synovial.
D the angle at which the thyroid laminae meet is greater in males than females.
E at birth, the body of the hyoid bone is usually ossified.

33 Regarding the thyroid gland:

A it receives all of its blood supply from the external carotid artery.
B the thyroidea ima artery is present in about 50% of cases.
C the inferior thyroid veins drain into the internal jugular vein.
D the carotid sheath is a posterolateral relation.
E the recurrent laryngeal nerve is a posteromedial relation.

34 With respect to the parathyroid glands:

A they are variable in number in the majority of individuals.
B the superior glands are more constant in position than the inferior glands.
C the inferior glands arise from the fourth pharyngeal pouch.
D they receive most of their blood supply from the inferior thyroid artery.
E normal parathyroid tissue may be located in the superior mediastinum.

31 A False The corniculate and cuneiform cartilages, and the epiglottis are fibrocartilage and do not ossify. The thyroid, cricoid and arytenoid cartilages are hyaline cartilage and commonly ossify

B True

C False The laryngeal ventricle separates the true and false cords.

D True

E True

32 A True

B False The thyroid cartilage is at C4; the cricoid cartilage is at C6.

C True The cricothyroid articulation is also synovial.

D False The laminae meet at an angle of approximately 90° in males and 120° in females, i.e. males have a greater laryngeal prominence.

E True The body and greater horn of the hyoid ossify at birth. The lesser horn ossifies during adolescence.

33 A False The blood supply is from the external carotid artery (superior thyroid branch) and from the thyrocervical trunk (inferior thyroid artery).

B False The thyroidea ima artery is present in about 3% of cases. It enters the lower border of the thyroid isthmus either from the brachiocephalic trunk, or directly from the aortic arch.

C False The superior and middle thyroid veins drain into the internal jugular vein. The inferior thyroid vein drains into the innominate vein.

D True

E True

34 A False About 90% of individuals have four parathyroid glands, 2.5% have five glands.

B True

C False The inferior parathyroid glands arise from the third pharyngeal pouch. The superior parathyroid glands arise from the fourth pharyngeal pouch.

D True

E True

35   The female breast:
A   lies on the deep fascia of the anterior chest wall between the second and sixth ribs.
B   is supported by the ligaments of Cooper.
C   has about 50 main ducts.
D   has its exocrine tissue replaced by fat with increasing age.
E   obtains its entire blood supply from the lateral thoracic artery.

36   Regarding the pericardium:
A   it comprises two layers between which is a potential space containing 20–25 ml serous fluid.
B   it extends to surround the entire length of the superior vena cava.
C   it is normally 1–2 mm thick.
D   the transverse sinus lies behind the ascending aorta.
E   the oesophagus is an immediate posterior relation.

37   In the heart:
A   the right atrium is the most posterior chamber.
B   the crista terminalis separates the right atrium from its appendage.
C   the left ventricle is characterised by a muscular conus (or infundibulum) and trabeculae carnae.
D   the left atrium receives two pulmonary veins.
E   the left ventricle is the most anterior chamber.

38   Regarding the heart valves:
A   in the normal individual, the mitral valve is the only bicuspid valve.
B   on the frontal projection the aortic valve is the only valve that lies to the right of the midline.
C   In the lateral projection the pulmonary valve is the most anterior of the valves.
D   In the lateral projection the mitral valve is the most inferior of the valves.
E   The competence of the atrioventricular valves is reinforced by chordae tendinae.

35 A **True**
    B **True**   These ligaments are fibrous tissue strands.
    C **False**   The breast has about 15 main ducts, each of which
                      drains a lobe of the breast, and opens onto the nipple.
    D **True**
    E **False**   The blood supply to the breast is derived mainly
                      from the lateral thoracic artery, but it also receives
                      branches from the internal mammary and intercostal
                      arteries.

36 A **True**   The two layers are the fibrous and the serous
                      pericardium.
    B **False**   Only the part of the superior vena cava below the
                      azygos vein insertion is enveloped by pericardium.
    C **True**
    D **True**   The transverse sinus is a pericardial recess which
                      may be mistaken for mediastinal adenopathy. The
                      superior recess or oblique sinus lies in front of the
                      aorta.
    E **True**

37 A **False**   The left atrium is the most posterior chamber.
    B **True**   The crista terminalis is a muscular ridge on the
                      posterior wall of the right atrium, between the
                      superior and inferior vena cava.
    C **False**   These features characterise the right ventricle, aiding
                      easy recognition at angiography.
    D **False**   The left atrium receives four pulmonary veins.
    E **False**   The right ventricle is the most anterior chamber.

38 A **True**   The aortic, pulmonary and tricuspid valves each have
                      three cusps.
    B **False**   The tricuspid valve is the only valve lying to the right
                      of the midline.
    C **True**
    D **False**   The tricuspid valve is the most inferior of the four
                      valves.
    E **True**   The chordae are attached to the free borders of the
                      cusps and to papillary muscles which arise from the
                      ventricular walls.

39   Regarding the coronary arteries:
A   the right coronary artery arises from the right posterior aortic sinus.
B   the sinoatrial node is usually supplied by the right coronary artery.
C   approximately 90% of individuals show right coronary artery dominance.
D   the circumflex artery has several diagonal branches.
E   the left anterior descending artery runs in the atrioventricular groove.

40   With respect to the venous drainage of the heart:
A   the coronary sinus receives about 90% of the venous drainage.
B   the coronary sinus lies in the posterior atrioventricular groove.
C   the coronary sinus drains directly into the right atrium.
D   the anterior cardiac veins drain into the coronary sinus.
E   the great cardiac vein accompanies the posterior interventricular artery.

41   Regarding the diaphragm:
A   the left crus is longer than the right.
B   the left hemidiaphragm is usually higher than the right.
C   the oesophageal hiatus passes through the central tendon.
D   the medial arcuate ligament is a thickening of the psoas fascia.
E   the aorta passes posterior to the median arcuate ligament accompanied by the thoracic duct and azygos vein.

39 A False   The right coronary artery arises from the anterior aortic sinus. The left coronary artery arises from the left posterior aortic sinus.

B True   The sinoatrial node is supplied by the right coronary artery in about 60% of cases. The atrioventricular node is supplied by the right coronary artery in about 90% of cases.

C True   The dominant artery is defined as that giving off the posterior interventricular branch.

D False   The diagonal branches arise from the left anterior descending artery. The circumflex artery has a left marginal branch.

E False   The circumflex branch of the left coronary artery runs in the atrioventricular groove posteriorly. The left anterior descending artery runs in the interventricular groove.

40 A False   The coronary sinus receives 60% of the venous drainage.

B True

C True

D False   The anterior cardiac veins and venae cordis minimae open directly into the right atrium. The great cardiac, middle cardiac and small cardiac veins drain into the coronary sinus.

E False   The great cardiac vein accompanies the left anterior descending artery in the interventricular groove. The middle cardiac vein accompanies the posterior interventricular artery in the posterior interventricular groove.

41 A False   The right is longer. It attaches to L1–3, whereas the left attaches to L1 and L2 only.

B False   The right hemidiaphragm is 1.5–2.5 cm higher than the left in 90% of cases.

C False   The oesophageal hiatus passes through the crura of the diaphragm at the level of T10. The hiatus for the inferior vena cava is through the central tendon (level T8).

D True

E True   The aortic opening is at the T12 level.

42 Concerning the peritoneal spaces:
  A the right paracolic gutter communicates directly with the right subhepatic space.
  B the left paracolic gutter communicates directly with the left subphrenic space.
  C Rutherford Morison's pouch is the most dependent part of the right paravertebral groove in a supine patient.
  D the lesser sac is related posteriorly to the right kidney.
  E the lesser sac is related anteriorly to the stomach.

43 Regarding the normal duodenum:
  A the first part begins to the left of L2.
  B the first part is completely retroperitoneal.
  C the accessory pancreatic duct opens into the second part distal to the duodenal papilla.
  D valvulae conniventes are absent in the fourth part.
  E the first part may be indented by the gall bladder.

44 Regarding the duodenum:
  A the first part lies anterior to the gastroduodenal artery.
  B the first part lies posterior to the gall bladder and the quadrate lobe of the liver.
  C the second part lies anterior to the left kidney.
  D the third part lies anterior to the superior mesenteric vessels.
  E the paraduodenal fossa lies to the left of the fourth part of the duodenum.

42 **A** **True**   The right paracolic gutter also communicates with
the right subphrenic space.

   B **False**   This communication is prevented by the
phrenicocolic ligament extending from the splenic
flexure of the colon to the left hemidiaphragm.

   C **True**   Rutherford Morison's pouch, the hepatorenal fossa, is
the posterior extension of the right subhepatic space.

   D **False**   The lesser sac is related posteriorly to the left kidney,
left adrenal, pancreas and left hemidiaphragm.

   E **True**   The lesser sac is related anteriorly to the lesser
omentum, stomach and greater omentum.

41 **A** **False**   The duodenum begins at the pylorus which lies
about 2 cm to the right of L1. It ends at the
duodenojejunal flexure which lies to the left of L2.

   B **False**   The first 2 cm of the first part of the duodenum has a
short mesentery.

   C **False**   The accessory pancreatic duct lies anterosuperior to
the duodenal papilla.

   D **False**   Valvulae conniventes begin in the second part of the
duodenum, becoming more prominent distally.

   E **True**

44 **A** **True**   It also lies anterior to the common bile duct.

   B **True**

   C **False**   The second part of the duodenum lies anterior to the
hilum of the right kidney and renal vessels. It lies
posterior to the transverse mesocolon.

   D **False**   The third part is crossed anteriorly by the superior
mesenteric vessels and the root of the small bowel
mesentery. It passes to the left anterior to the inferior
vena cava and abdominal aorta at the level of L3.

   E **True**   The paraduodenal fossa is a recess of peritoneum
beneath the most cephalad part of the inferior
mesenteric vein.

45 The following statements are true:
  A the superior mesenteric artery is retroperitoneal.
  B the jejunum has a maximum diameter of approximately 4 cm.
  C the valvulae conniventes are about 1 mm thick in the middle and distal ileum.
  D a Meckel's diverticulum is present in about 2% of people.
  E the stomach receives branches from the common hepatic artery.

46 In the large bowel:
  A the appendix is retrocaecal in the majority of cases.
  B there is a sigmoid mesentery.
  C the ileocaecal valve lies anteromedially in the majority of cases.
  D the taeniae coli converge on the ileocaecal valve.
  E the haustra are more clearly defined in the ascending colon than in the descending colon.

45 A False   It lies within the mesentery.
    B True   The Ileum has a smaller maximum diameter (approximately 3 cm).
    C True   They are thicker in the jejunum, where they measure approximately 2 mm. They may be absent in the distended terminal ileum.
    D True   This remnant of the vitellointestinal duct is usually located in the ileum within 1 m of the ileocaecal valve. It typically measures less than 5 cm in length.
    E True   The stomach receives part of its blood supply from the right gastric and gastroduodenal arteries. Both are branches of the common hepatic artery.

---

46 A True   It is retrocaecal in approximately 64% of cases.
    B True   The mesentery starts at the rectosigmoid junction, usually at the level of S3.
    C False   It lies posteromedially in approximately 90% of cases, in line with the first complete transverse haustral cleft of the proximal colon.
    D False   The taeniae coli, one anterior, one posteromedial and one posterolateral, converge on the base of the appendix.
    E True   The haustral sacculations arise between the three rows of taeniae, with clefts at the points of circular muscle fusion. In the proximal colon the haustra are fixed, whereas they result from active contraction of the taeniae from the mid-transverse colon onwards. When smooth muscle relaxants are given during a double-contrast barium enema, the left colon often shows no haustration.

47 **The rectum:**
   A   is filled by air during a double contrast barium enema when
       the patient lies prone.
   B   is covered by the peritoneum anteriorly and laterally in its
       upper two thirds.
   C   has lateral crescentic folds (plicae semilunares) which consist
       of mucosa and submucosa.
   D   has venous drainage to the portal system only.
   E   receives its main blood supply from the inferior mesenteric
       artery.

48 **The abdominal aorta:**
   A   bifurcates at the level of L5.
   B   gives rise to the coeliac axis at the level of T12.
   C   gives rise to four paired lumbar arteries.
   D   gives rise to the inferior phrenic arteries.
   E   is crossed anteriorly by the left renal vein at the level of L2.

49 **The inferior vena cava:**
   A   is longer than the aorta within the abdomen.
   B   drains the median sacral veins.
   C   drains the right adrenal and gonadal veins directly.
   D   is partly derived from the right supracardinal vein.
   E   is left sided in approximately 0.5% of cases.

47 **A** **True**

    B **False** Pelvic peritoneum covers the upper third of the rectum anteriorly and laterally, the middle third anteriorly only and the lower third not at all.

    C **True** There are usually three lateral crescentic folds, less than 5 mm thick, but they are variable in configuration.

    D **False** The superior rectal vein drains into the portal system whilst the middle and inferior rectal veins drain into the systemic venous system. The rectum therefore forms a site of porto-caval anastomosis.

    E **True** It also receives blood from the middle rectal branches of the internal iliac arteries, the inferior rectal branches of the internal pudendal arteries and the median sacral artery.

48 **A** **False** It bifurcates at the level of the body of L4.

    B **True** It gives rise to the superior mesenteric and inferior mesenteric arteries at the L1 and L3 levels respectively.

    C **True**

    D **True** The aorta also gives rise to paired visceral branches: the adrenal, renal and gonadal arteries. The median sacral artery also arises from its posterior surface at the bifurcation.

    E **True**

49 **A** **True** The inferior vena cava starts at the level of L5, lower than the bifurcation of the aorta, and passes through the central tendon of the diaphragm at T8 (four vertebrae higher than the commencement of the abdominal aorta).

    B **False** The median sacral veins, companions to the artery, drain into the left common iliac vein in front of the body of L5.

    C **True** Whereas the left adrenal and gonadal veins enter the left renal vein. The inferior vena cava also receives drainage direct from both renal veins, the third and fourth lumbar veins, the hepatic veins and the inferior phrenic veins.

    D **True** The inferior vena cava is derived from the persisting right supracardinal, right subcardinal and right vitelline veins.

    E **True** The left inferior vena cava drains the left renal vein, crosses the spine and continues cranially as a normal right-sided inferior vena cava.

50 The superior mesenteric artery:
A   anastomoses with the inferior mesenteric artery at the hepatic flexure.
B   supplies the left lobe of the liver in about 40% of cases.
C   gives rise to the inferior pancreaticoduodenal artery.
D   lies to the left of the superior mesenteric vein.
E   passes anterior to the left renal vein.

51 The spleen:
A   lies along the line of the eighth rib.
B   lies on the phrenicocolic ligament.
C   is directly related to the left kidney.
D   receives its blood supply via the gastrosplenic ligament.
E   may normally indent the greater curve of the stomach.

52 The pancreas:
A   decreases in size with advancing age.
B   lies anterior to the confluence of the superior mesenteric and splenic veins.
C   originates entirely from the dorsal gut diverticulum.
D   is retroperitoneal.
E   has a main duct which measures approximately 6 mm in diameter.

50 A False The left branch of the middle colic artery (of the superior mesenteric artery) anastomoses with a branch of the left colic artery (of the inferior mesenteric artery) in the region of the splenic flexure.

B False The left hepatic artery arises from the superior mesenteric artery in about 4% of cases.

C True The inferior pancreaticoduodenal artery is the first branch of the superior mesenteric artery. It anastomoses with the superior pancreaticoduodenal artery, a branch of the gastroduodenal artery.

D True

E True The superior mesenteric artery passes anterior to the left renal vein and the third part of the duodenum to enter the mesentery of the small intestine.

51 A False Its long axis lies along the line of the tenth rib.

B True

C True The spleen abuts the upper pole of the left kidney. This produces a prominence on the lateral aspect of the kidney.

D False The splenic artery enters the spleen via the splenorenal ligament, which also contains the splenic vein and pancreatic tail.

E True The spleen is related anteriorly to the greater curve of the stomach and the splenic flexure of the colon, which both show splenic impressions.

52 A True Pancreatic tissue is gradually replaced by fat and fibrous tissue with advancing age.

B True The pancreatic neck lies anterior to this venous confluence.

C False The uncinate process and part of the pancreatic head develop from the ventral gut diverticulum. The remainder of the pancreatic head, body and tail develop from the dorsal diverticulum.

D True

E False The calibre of the main pancreatic duct increases with age, but in subjects younger than 60 years, its maximum diameter in the region of the body should be no more than 2 mm.

53   The head of the pancreas:

    A is more cephalad than the tail.

    B lies anterior to the common bile duct.

    C is drained by the main pancreatic duct of Wirsung.

    D receives its main blood supply from branches of the splenic artery.

    E has an uncinate process which is crossed by the superior mesenteric vessels.

54   The gall bladder:

    A usually has a volume of approximately 300 ml.

    B is related to the hepatic flexure of the colon.

    C has a spiral valve composed of smooth muscle.

    D normally has a wall thickness of about 1 cm.

    E typically lies anteromedial to the right lobe of the liver.

55   In the liver:

    A a Riedel's lobe is more common in males than in females.

    B venous drainage of the quadrate lobe is usually distinct from the rest of the liver.

    C the ligamentum teres is a remnant of the umbilical vein.

    D the caudate lobe lies between the inferior vena cava and the porta hepatis.

    E the bare area of the liver is applied directly to the diaphragm.

53 **A** **False** The tail of the pancreas is higher than the head.
    B **True** It also lies anterior to the inferior vena cava in the region of the termination of the renal veins.

    C **True**
    D **False** It receives its main blood supply from pancreaticoduodenal arcades formed by branches of the gastroduodenal and superior mesenteric arteries. The neck, body and tail of the pancreas receive their main blood supply from branches of the splenic artery.

    E **True**

---

54 **A** **False** The volume of the gall bladder is usually about 30–50 ml.

    B **True**
    C **False** The spiral valve (of Heister) in the neck of the gall bladder is composed of crescentic folds of mucosa.

    D **False** The normal gall bladder wall thickness is about 1 mm.
    E **True**

---

55 **A** **False** A Riedel's lobe, the downward projection of the anterolateral aspect of the right lobe of the liver, is more common in females.

    B **False** The venous drainage of the caudate lobe is frequently distinct from the rest of the liver, direct to the inferior vena cava, rather than into the hepatic veins.

    C **True** It runs in the free edge of the falciform ligament which extends from the umbilicus.

    D **True** Whereas the quadrate lobe lies inferiorly and is bordered by the ligamentum teres and the gall bladder. Both the caudate lobe and the quadrate lobe are segments of the left lobe of the liver.

    E **True** The bare area contains part of the inferior vena cava and hepatic veins.

56 In the hepatobiliary system:
   A the cystic artery arises from the right hepatic artery in the
      majority of cases.
   B the cystic duct usually lies to the left of the common hepatic
      duct.
   C the right hepatic artery crosses dorsal to the portal vein in
      about 10% of cases.
   D the right portal vein receives blood mainly from the superior
      mesenteric vein.
   E the hepatic veins follow the structures of the portal triad.

57 The portal vein:
   A lies posterior to the common bile duct.
   B is formed by the union of the splenic and inferior mesenteric
      veins.
   C receives the left gastric vein.
   D receives the right colic vein.
   E provides about 75% of the blood supply to the liver.

58 Regarding the adrenal glands:
   A the medial limb of the right adrenal gland is smaller than the
      lateral limb.
   B the right adrenal gland lies cephalad to the right kidney.
   C the right crus of the diaphragm is a medial relation of the right
      adrenal gland.
   D they receive branches from the inferior phrenic arteries.
   E the left adrenal vein drains directly into the inferior vena cava.

56 **A** **True**   In about 90% of cases.

    B **False**   It usually lies on the right of the common hepatic duct.

    C **True**   In the large majority of cases the right hepatic artery crosses ventral to the portal vein.

    D **True**   Whereas the left portal vein receives blood mainly from the splenic and inferior mesenteric veins.

    E **False**   The hepatic veins are intersegmental, in that they drain portions of adjacent segments of the liver and converge on the inferior vena cava. Each segment of the liver is supplied by a portal triad (hepatic artery, bile duct and portal vein).

57 **A** **True**   In the free edge of the lesser omentum the common bile duct lies to the right, the hepatic artery to the left and the portal vein posteriorly. At the porta hepatis, the arrangement is: duct, artery and vein from anterior to posterior.

    B **False**   The portal vein is formed behind the neck of the pancreas by the union of the splenic and superior mesenteric veins, with the inferior mesenteric vein joining at or near the angle of this union.

    C **True**   The portal vein usually also receives the right gastric vein, cystic vein and some duodenal or pancreatic veins.

    D **False**   The right colic vein drains into the superior mesenteric vein, along with the right gastroepiploic, pancreaticoduodenal, jejunal, ileal and middle colic veins.

    E **True**   25% of the blood supply to the liver is provided by the hepatic arteries.

58 **A** **False**   The lateral limb of the right adrenal gland is the smaller.

    B **True**   The left adrenal gland lies anterior to the upper pole of the left kidney.

    C **True**

    D **True**   Superior adrenal branches arise from the inferior phrenic arteries bilaterally. The adrenal glands are also supplied by the middle adrenal arteries, which are direct branches from the aorta, and the inferior adrenal arteries, which are branches of the renal arteries.

    E **False**   The left adrenal vein drains into the left renal vein. The right adrenal vein drains directly into the inferior vena cava at the level of T12.

59 The right adrenal gland is directly related to the:
    A quadrate lobe of the liver.
    B aorta.
    C body of the pancreas.
    D second part of the duodenum.
    E epiploic foramen.

60 Regarding the kidneys:
    A the renal artery lies posterior to the ureter at the hilum.
    B their superior poles lie closer to the median plane than their inferior poles.
    C about 25% of kidneys receive their blood supply via multiple aortic branches.
    D both are related to the colon anteriorly.
    E typically each renal artery divides into four segmental branches.

61 The right kidney:
    A is usually smaller than the left.
    B usually lies lower than the left.
    C usually moves further during respiration than the left.
    D is related to the duodenum.
    E is drained by the right renal vein which is longer than the left renal vein.

62 Each ureter:
    A has three narrowings along its length.
    B is lined by transitional cell epithelium.
    C is retroperitoneal.
    D lies lateral to the tips of the transverse processes of the lumbar vertebrae.
    E receives part of its blood supply from the gonadal arteries.

59 **A** **False** The right adrenal gland is related to the bare area of the liver.

    B **False** The right adrenal gland is related to the inferior vena cava.

    C **False** The left adrenal gland is related to the body of the pancreas.

    D **False** The second part of the duodenum is separated from the right adrenal gland by the inferior vena cava.

    E **False** The inferior vena cava lies between the epiploic foramen and the right adrenal gland.

60 **A** **False** At the renal hilum, the renal vein lies anteriorly, the ureter posteriorly and the renal artery in between.

    B **True**

    C **True** There may be two, three or four renal arteries which enter through the renal sinus or at the superior or inferior pole of the kidney.

    D **True** Anteriorly the right and left kidneys are related to the hepatic and splenic flexures of the colon respectively.

    E **False** The renal artery typically divides into posterior and anterior branches, which together supply five segments: apical and posterior (from the posterior branch) and anterosuperior, anteroinferior and inferior (from the anterior branch).

61 **A** **True**

    B **True**

    C **False** The left kidney moves further than the right.

    D **True** The duodenum is related to the anterior surface of the right kidney.

    E **False** The left renal vein is longer than the right, crossing the aorta anteriorly to open into the inferior vena cava superior to the right renal vein.

62 **A** **True** These narrowings occur at the pelviureteric junction, pelvic brim and vesicoureteric junction.

    B **True**

    C **True**

    D **False** The ureters lie medial to the tips of the transverse processes of the lumbar vertebrae.

    E **True** The ureters receive their blood supply from branches of the renal, gonadal, common iliac and vesical arteries.

63   The right ureter lies:

A   anterior to the iliac vessels.
B   posterior to the gonadal vessels.
C   posterior to the ileocolic artery.
D   inferior to the vas deferens in the male pelvis.
E   inferior to the broad ligament in the female pelvis.

64   Regarding the bony pelvis:

A   the inferior portion of the sacroiliac joint is synovial.
B   the subpubic angle in the adult female is greater than that in the male.
C   the symphysis pubis is a synovial joint.
D   the sacrum usually consists of four fused vertebrae with five paired anterior sacral foramina.
E   the adductor magnus muscle arises from the ischiopubic ramus and ischial tuberosity.

65   The right ischiorectal fossa:

A   has part of its lateral wall formed by the obturator externus muscle.
B   contains the pudendal canal on its lateral wall.
C   does not communicate with the left ischiorectal fossa.
D   has part of its medial wall formed by the levator ani muscle.
E   contains fat.

66   In adults the normal size of:

A   the nulliparous uterus is approximately 4 cm × 2 cm.
B   the testis is approximately 4 cm × 2.5 cm.
C   the prostate is approximately 8 cm × 10 cm.
D   the ovary is approximately 0.2 cm × 0.3 cm × 0.4 cm.
E   the internal cervical os is up to 6 mm in diameter.

63 **A** **True**
   B **True**
   C **True**   The right ureter lies posterior to the ileocolic and right colic vessels, and the duodenum and the small bowel mesentery. The left ureter lies posterior to the left colic vessels and the sigmoid mesentery.
   D **True**
   E **True**

---

64 **A** **True**   The superior portion of the sacroiliac joint is fibrous.
   B **True**   The subpubic angle is about 85° and 55° in the adult female and male pelves respectively.
   C **False**   The symphysis pubis is a secondary cartilaginous joint.
   D **False**   The sacrum usually consists of five fused vertebrae with four paired anterior sacral foramina.
   E **True**

---

65 **A** **False**   The lateral wall of the ischiorectal fossa is formed by the ischial tuberosity below and the obturator internus muscle above.
   B **True**
   C **False**   The fossae communicate with each other through loose tissue behind the anal canal providing a horseshoe-shaped path for the spread of infection.
   D **True**   The anal canal and levator ani muscles form the medial wall of each fossa.
   E **True**   The ischiorectal fat pad allows for dilatation of the anal canal during defaecation and of the vagina during parturition.

---

66 **A** **False**   The non-pregnant uterus normally measures approximately 8 cm × 5 cm.
   B **True**
   C **False**   The prostate is approximately 3 cm long and 4 cm wide.
   D **False**   The normal dimensions of the adult ovary are 2 cm × 3 cm × 4 cm.
   E **True**

67 Regarding the uterus:
- A   the pouch of Douglas is an anterior relation.
- B   the paired round ligaments are folds of peritoneum.
- C   the arterial supply is from the internal iliac artery.
- D   it is covered by peritoneum on all but the inferior surface.
- E   the isthmus is in continuity with the cervix.

68 Regarding the fallopian tubes:
- A   each tube is approximately 10 cm long.
- B   they communicate with the peritoneal cavity.
- C   they lie in the inferior border of the broad ligament.
- D   the isthmus is the narrowest segment.
- E   the folds of mucous membrane are arranged in the most complex manner in the region of the ampulla.

69 Regarding the ovaries:
- A   prior to ovulation follicles measure approximately 18–24 mm.
- B   venous drainage of the right ovary is to the right renal vein.
- C   they lie anterolateral to the uterus.
- D   they commonly calcify in normal individuals.
- E   they lie anterior to the ureters.

67 A False   The pouch of Douglas (rectouterine pouch) lies
                   posterior to the uterus.
B False   The round ligaments support the uterus and
                   comprise fibromuscular bands extending from the
                   labium majorum, through the deep inguinal ring to
                   attach to the uterus. The broad ligaments are folds of
                   peritoneum.
C True
D True
E True   The isthmus is the lowest half centimetre of the body
                   of the uterus and this is continuous with the cervix.

68 A True
B True
C False   The uterine tubes lie in the superior border of the
                   broad ligament.
D True   The other segments of the uterine tube are: the
                   uterine, ampulla and infundibulum.
E True   The uterine tubes are lined with mucous membrane
                   which is arranged in folds which are sparse in the
                   isthmus and become increasingly complicated
                   towards the ampulla.

69 A True
B False   Venous drainage of the right ovary is to the inferior
                   vena cava. Venous drainage of the left ovary is to the
                   left renal vein.
C False   They lie posterolateral to the uterus.
D False   Physiological calcification is rarely visible in the
                   corpus albicans.
E True

70   In antenatal ultrasound:

A   the fetal heart is first detectable at 4 weeks gestation.
B   the crown-rump length is the best measurement for assessing maturity at 6–12 weeks gestation.
C   the normal biparietal diameter at 18 weeks is approximately 40 mm.
D   the lateral ventricular ratio should not exceed 35%.
E   the gut is normally extra-abdominal at 16 weeks gestation.

71   The testis:

A   has the epididymis as an immediate posterolateral relation.
B   is surrounded by a fibrous capsule called the tunica vaginalis.
C   has its venous drainage to the internal iliac vein.
D   contains the rete testis near its posterior border.
E   usually lies within the scrotum by the seventh fetal month.

72   The vas deferens:

A   is embryologically derived from the Wolffian duct.
B   commences at the head of the epididymis.
C   is extraperitoneal within the pelvis.
D   at the ampulla, lies medial to the seminal vesicles.
E   loops over the ureter as the ureter enters the bladder.

70 **A** **False**   It is first detectable at 6–7 weeks gestation.
    B **True**   Biparietal diameter may be used to assess maturity at 12–30 weeks, femur length at 14–22 weeks and fetal abdominal circumference at 30–40 weeks.

    C **True**
    D **True**   The lateral ventricular ratio is calculated by dividing the distance from the midline to the lateral wall of the lateral ventricle by the distance from the midline to the inner table of the skull, in the coronal plane.

    E **False**   A loop of gut extrudes into the umbilical cord as the "physiological hernia" at about the end of the sixth week of gestation, and returns to the abdominal cavity towards the end of the tenth week.

---

71 **A** **True**
    B **False**   The tunica vaginalis is a serous sac covering the anterior and lateral surfaces of the testis. The tunica albuginea is a fibrous capsule.

    C **False**   Venous drainage of the testes is via the testicular veins. The right testicular vein drains to the inferior vena cava and the left to the left renal vein.

    D **True**   Semen drains via seminiferous tubules into the rete testis from where the vasa efferentia pass towards the epididymis.

    E **False**   By the seventh fetal month the testis lies at the deep inguinal ring. It should be in the scrotum by birth.

---

72 **A** **True**
    B **False**   Each vas deferens commences at the tail of the epididymis in the scrotum.

    C **True**
    D **True**
    E **True**

73 Regarding the male urethra:
A the membranous urethra is the widest part.
B the verumontanum is on the anterior wall of the prostatic urethra.
C the prostatic duct openings lie lateral to the verumontanum.
D the navicular fossa lies within the bulb of the urethra.
E the penile urethra lies within the corpus spongiosum of the penis.

74 Regarding the bladder:
A it has a capacity of approximately 1.5 l.
B the trigone lies between the ureteric orifices and the urethra.
C the seminal vesicles are posterior relations in the male.
D the obturator internus muscle is an inferolateral relation.
E the pubovesical ligaments support the bladder superiorly.

75 The following have their lymphatic drainage predominantly to the external iliac lymph nodes:
A testes.
B bladder.
C prostate.
D uterus.
E rectum.

76 Concerning the cranial foramina and canals:
A the superior orbital fissure transmits the maxillary division of the fifth cranial nerve.
B the foramen ovale transmits the mandibular division of the fifth cranial nerve.
C the foramen spinosum transmits the middle meningeal artery.
D the superior orbital fissure lies between the greater and lesser wings of the sphenoid.
E the left jugular foramen is usually larger than the right.

73 A **False**   The prostatic urethra is the widest part.
   B **False**   The verumontanum is on the posterior wall of the
               prostatic urethra and has the utricle and ejaculatory
               duct orifices on its ventral wall.
   C **True**
   D **False**   The navicular fossa is a short dilated region just
               proximal to the external urethral meatus.
   E **True**

74 A **False**   Capacity is about 500 ml.
   B **True**
   C **True**
   D **True**
   E **False**   The pubovesical ligaments are condensations of
               pelvic fascia that support the bladder inferiorly, along
               with puboprostatic ligaments in the male.

75 A **False**   The testes have their lymphatic drainage to the
               para-aortic lymph nodes.
   B **True**
   C **False**   The prostate has its lymphatic drainage to the
               internal iliac nodes and sacral nodes.
   D **True**
   E **False**   The rectum has its lymphatic drainage to the
               pararectal, preaortic and internal iliac nodes.

76 A **False**   The foramen rotundum transmits the maxillary
               nerve. The superior orbital fissure transmits the third,
               fourth and sixth cranial nerves, and the first branch
               of the fifth cranial nerve, along with the superior
               ophthalmic vein.
   B **True**
   C **True**
   D **True**
   E **False**   The right jugular foramen is often larger than the left.

77   Regarding the bones of the skull:
   A   the pterygoid processes arise from the inferior surface of the
       body of the sphenoid bone.
   B   the occipital bone forms the posterior half of the clivus.
   C   the occipital condyles are situated at the posterior half of the
       foramen magnum.
   D   the jugular foramen lies lateral to the hypoglossal canal.
   E   the internal jugular vein is transmitted through the medial
       portion of the jugular foramen.

78   Regarding grooves and sutures of the calvarium:
   A   the "parietal star" is caused by venous sinuses impressing on
       the inner table of the skull.
   B   parietal foramina are usually situated close to the sagittal
       suture.
   C   the bregma is the point where the sagittal suture meets the
       lambdoid suture.
   D   the asterion is the point where the lambdoid suture meets the
       squamosal suture.
   E   sutural sclerosis becomes more apparent with increasing age.

79   Regarding the skull in infancy and childhood:
   A   the metopic suture passes obliquely through the occipital bone.
   B   the metopic suture usually fuses within the first 6 months of
       extrauterine life.
   C   closure of the posterior fontanelle occurs at 18 months of age.
   D   at birth there are no vascular markings and no convolutional
       impressions.
   E   the spheno-occipital synchondrosis begins to close by the age
       of 5 years.

77 A **True**
    B **True**
    C **False** The occipital condyles lie at the anterior half of the foramen magnum, their posterior poles separated by the width of the foramen and their anterior poles lying closer together.
    D **True**
    E **False** The internal jugular vein is transmitted through the lateral portion of the jugular foramen. The ninth, tenth and eleventh cranial nerves pass through the medial portion of the jugular foramen.

78 A **False** The "parietal star" is caused by venous plexuses lying between the inner and outer tables of the skull.
    B **True**
    C **False** The lambda marks the junction of the sagittal and lambdoid sutures. The bregma marks the junction of the sagittal and coronal sutures.
    D **True** The pterion marks the point where the coronal suture meets the sphenoid bone laterally.
    E **True** Sutural sclerosis is a physiological bony bridging process across the suture.

79 A **False** The mendosal sutures pass obliquely upwards and inwards from the lower part of the occipital bone bilaterally.
    B **False** The metopic suture of the frontal bone is present at birth, disappears from the ninth month onwards and is usually fused by the end of the second year. Occasionally it persists into adult life.
    C **False** Closure of the posterior fontanelle usually occurs at 6–8 months. Closure of the anterior fontanelle usually occurs at 15–18 months.
    D **True** The vascular markings and convolutional impressions appear between the second and third years.
    E **False** The spheno-occipital synchondrosis begins to close during puberty.

80   The following may be seen on a submentovertical (axial) projection of the skull:

A   the foramen spinosum.
B   the lateral wall of the maxillary antrum.
C   the odontoid process of the axis.
D   the dorsum sellae.
E   the carotid canal.

81   The following may be seen on a half-axial (Towne's) projection of the skull:

A   the foramen ovale.
B   the foramen rotundum.
C   the internal auditory meati.
D   the superior orbital fissure.
E   the condyle of the mandible.

82   Physiological intracranial calcification occurs in:

A   the pineal gland in approximately 5% of adults.
B   the habenular commissure.
C   the petroclinoid ligaments.
D   the falx cerebri.
E   the diaphragma sellae.

83   Regarding the branches of the aortic arch:

A   the common carotid artery bifurcates at about the level of the second cervical vertebra.
B   in the neck, the internal carotid artery lies medial to the external carotid artery throughout its length.
C   the left common carotid artery arises from the innominate artery in about 27% of cases.
D   an aberrant right subclavian artery occurs in about 1% of the population.
E   the left common carotid and left subclavian arteries have a common origin in about 1% of cases.

80 A **True**
    B **True**   The lateral wall of the maxillary antrum has an
                     S-shaped configuration which is superimposed on
                     the lateral wall of the orbit; the latter appearing as a
                     straight line.
    C **True**
    D **False**   The dorsum sellae is seen on lateral and half-axial
                     (Towne's) projections.
    E **True**

81 A **False**   The foramen ovale is best seen on the
                     submentovertical projection.
    B **False**   The foramen rotundum is best seen on the
                     occipitofrontal projection.
    C **True**
    D **False**   The superior orbital fissure is best seen on the
                     occipitofrontal projection.
    E **True**

82 A **False**   It occurs in about 60% of adults.
    B **True**   In about 30% of adults.
    C **True**   In about 12% of adults.
    D **True**   In about 7% of adults.
    E **True**

83 A **False**   The common carotid artery divides into the external
                     and internal carotid arteries at about the level of the
                     fourth cervical vertebra.
    B **False**   The internal carotid artery lies posterior to the
                     external carotid artery; initially lateral to, and then
                     medial to it.
    C **True**   This is the most common normal variant affecting
                     the arteries arising from the aortic arch.
    D **True**
    E **True**

84   The following arteries arise directly from the internal carotid artery:

A   the meningohypophyseal artery.
B   the anterior communicating artery.
C   the callosomarginal artery.
D   the posterior communicating artery.
E   the ophthalmic artery.

85   Regarding the internal carotid artery:

A   it usually has no main branches in the neck.
B   on entering the cranial cavity, it becomes subarachnoid in position.
C   the carotid siphon is formed by the cavernous segment only.
D   it gives rise to the anterior choroidal artery.
E   it anastomoses with both the external carotid and vertebrobasilar arterial systems.

86   The external carotid artery gives rise to:

A   the ascending pharyngeal artery.
B   the inferior thyroid artery.
C   the internal maxillary artery.
D   the occipital artery.
E   the posterior auricular artery.

84 A True   The meningohypophyseal artery arises posteriorly within the cavernous sinus.

**   B False**   The anterior communicating artery acts as an arterial bridge between the anterior cerebral arteries. The latter are direct branches of the internal carotid arteries.

**   C False**   The callosomarginal artery is one of the three main branches of the anterior cerebral artery, distal to the anterior communicating artery. The other distal branches of the anterior cerebral artery are the frontopolar and pericallosal arteries.

**   D True**   The posterior communicating artery arises posteriorly from the distal loop of the carotid siphon to link the internal carotid artery with the posterior cerebral artery.

**   E True**   The ophthalmic artery is usually given off just after the carotid artery leaves the cavernous sinus; but its origin is variable.

---

85 A True

**   B False**   It lies external to the dura mater within the cranial cavity and cavernous sinus, and enters the subarachnoid space at the level of the anterior clinoid process.

**   C False**   The carotid siphon is formed by the cavernous and supraclinoid segments of the internal carotid artery.

**   D True**   The anterior choroidal artery arises posteriorly from the carotid siphon just distal to the posterior communicating artery.

**   E True**

---

86 A True

**   B False**   The inferior thyroid artery arises from the thyrocervical trunk which arises from the subclavian artery. The superior thyroid artery is usually the first branch of the external carotid artery, but may arise from the terminal part of the common carotid artery.

**   C True**   The internal maxillary artery is one of the terminal branches of the external carotid artery; as is the superficial temporal artery.

**   D True**

**   E True**   The external carotid artery also gives rise to the lingual and facial arteries.

87   The vertebral artery:

A   usually has a wider calibre on the left than the right.
B   usually enters the foramen transversarium of the seventh cervical vertebra.
C   arises from the thyrocervical trunk in some individuals.
D   is usually the first branch of the subclavian artery.
E   usually gives off the posterior inferior cerebellar artery just before entering the foramen magnum.

88   The cavernous sinus:

A   drains the ophthalmic veins.
B   drains into the superior and inferior petrosal sinuses.
C   contains the mandibular division of the trigeminal nerve.
D   lies lateral to the sphenoid sinus and pituitary fossa.
E   lies in the subarachnoid space.

89   Regarding the cerebral veins:

A   the septal vein and the thalamostriate vein join to form the great cerebral vein of Galen.
B   the great cerebral vein of Galen joins the inferior sagittal sinus to form the sigmoid sinus.
C   the superior sagittal sinus usually drains to the right transverse sinus.
D   the great cerebral vein of Galen lies in the quadrigeminal cistern.
E   the cavernous sinus communicates with the veins of the face.

87 **A** **True**   The left vertebral artery is usually the larger, but the right is larger in about 20% of cases.

B **False**   The vertebral artery usually passes through the foramina transversaria of the upper six cervical vertebrae. It enters the foramen of the seventh cervical vertebra in about 1% of cases.

C **True**
D **True**
E **False**   The vertebral artery gives off the posterior inferior cerebellar artery after entering the cranial cavity.

88 **A** **True**
B **True**
C **False**   The third, fourth and ophthalmic and maxillary divisions of the fifth cranial nerves lie in the lateral wall of the cavernous sinus. The sixth cranial nerve runs through the cavernous sinus inferior and lateral to the internal carotid artery. The mandibular nerve passes downwards through the foramen ovale into the infratemporal fossa.

D **True**
E **False**   The cavernous sinus lies between the layers of the dura mater.

89 **A** **False**   The septal vein and the thalamostriate vein join at the venous angle to form the internal cerebral vein. The internal cerebral veins and basal veins of Rosenthal join to form the great cerebral vein of Galen.

B **False**   The great cerebral vein joins the inferior sagittal sinus to form the straight sinus.

C **True**   The superior sagittal sinus usually becomes the right transverse sinus, the right sigmoid sinus, then the right internal jugular vein. The straight sinus drains in a similar sequence on the left side.

D **True**
E **True**   Via the ophthalmic veins and pterygoid plexus.

90   Regarding the ventricles of the brain:
  A   the interventricular foramen connects the third ventricle with the fourth ventricle.
  B   they communicate with the central canal of the spinal cord.
  C   the roof of the anterior horn of the lateral ventricle is formed by the corpus callosum.
  D   the pineal body lies in the posterior wall of the third ventricle.
  E   the median aperture (foramen of Magendie) connects the fourth ventricle with the cerebellomedullary cistern.

91   In the middle ear:
  A   the spur is formed by the junction of the external auditory canal and the lateral wall of the attic.
  B   the promontory forms the roof.
  C   the handle of the malleus is attached to the tympanic membrane.
  D   the incudomallear and incudostapedial joints are synovial.
  E   the ossicles have the appearance of a "molar tooth" on a lateral tomogram.

90 A False The interventricular foramina of Munro connect each lateral ventricle to the third ventricle. A midline channel, the cerebral aqueduct of Sylvius connects the third and fourth ventricles.

B True Below the fourth ventricle the central canal extends through the spinal cord into the upper end of the filum terminale.

C True The floor of the anterior horn of the lateral ventricle is formed by the caudate nucleus and thalamus.

D True The habenular commissure, pineal body and posterior commissure form the posterior wall of the third ventricle. The lamina terminalis forms the anterior wall and the thalamus forms most of the lateral walls. The hypothalamus forms the lower lateral wall and most of the floor.

E True Whereas the paired lateral apertures (foramina of Luschka) open into the pontine cistern. Through these three apertures, one median and two lateral, the cerebrospinal fluid escapes from the ventricular system into the subarachnoid space for absorption by the arachnoid villi.

91 A True This is also referred to as the scutum. It forms the superior attachment of the tympanic membrane.

B False The tegmen tympani forms the roof. The bony capsule of the basal turn of the cochlea is called the promontory.

C True

D True The incudomallear joint lies between the head of the malleus and the body of the incus. The incudostapedial joint lies between the long process of the incus and the head of the stapes.

E True The "crown" of the tooth is made up of the head of the malleus and the body of the incus. The "roots" of the tooth are the handle of the malleus and the long process of the incus. The malleus is anterior to the incus.

92 Regarding the ear:
  A   the second part of the facial canal lies inferior to the lateral
      semicircular canal.
  B   the carotid canal lies in the anterior wall of the middle ear.
  C   the oval window lies superior to the round window.
  D   the mastoid antrum lies posterior to the middle ear.
  E   the pyramid lies superior to the aditus to the antrum.

93 Regarding the paranasal sinuses:
  A   they are rudimentary in the neonatal skull.
  B   the frontal sinus opens into the superior meatus of the nasal
      cavity.
  C   the maxillary sinus opens into the middle meatus of the nasal
      cavity.
  D   they are lined by ciliated mucous columnar epithelium.
  E   the sphenoid sinus is usually divided into two by a thin
      septum.

94 In the temporomandibular joint:
  A   an articular disc divides the joint cavity into anterior and
      posterior compartments.
  B   the lateral pterygoid muscle is inserted partly into the articular
      disc.
  C   the capsule is attached inferiorly to the coronoid process of
      the mandible.
  D   the sphenomandibular ligament lies medially.
  E   stability is maximised by occlusion.

92 A True   The facial canal is divided into three parts. The first part, or genu, curves anteriorly adjacent to the cochlea and contains the geniculate ganglion. The second part doubles back posteriorly to lie beneath the lateral semicircular canal. The third part descends vertically posterior to the external auditory canal to emerge at the stylomastoid foramen.

   B True

   C True

   D True   The opening into the antrum, aditus to the antrum, lies in the superomedial part of the posterior wall of the middle ear.

   E False   The pyramid is a bony projection from the posterior wall of the middle ear, lying below the aditus, and giving rise to the stapedius muscle.

93 A True   The sinuses develop during childhood; the maxillary and ethmoid developing earlier than the frontal and sphenoid sinuses.

   B False   The frontal sinus opens into the middle meatus by the frontonasal duct.

   C True   In addition, the sphenoid sinus opens into the spheno-ethmoidal recess. The anterior and middle ethmoidal air cells open into the middle meatus and the posterior ethmoidal air cells into the superior meatus.

   D True

   E True

94 A False   The fibrocartilaginous articular disc divides the joint cavity into superior and inferior compartments which allow sliding and rotational movements respectively.

   B True   The lateral pterygoid muscle passes through the capsule of the joint to be inserted into the disc.

   C False   The capsule is attached inferiorly to the neck of the condylar process of the mandible.

   D True   The sphenomandibular ligament passes from the spine of the sphenoid to the lingula of the mandible.

   E True   The joint is less stable in the open position.

95 Regarding dentition:

A   the normal adult has 32 teeth.

B   there are normally 20 deciduous teeth.

C   the periodontal membrane is seen as a radiodense line outlining the root of a tooth on a radiograph.

D   enamel is the most radiopaque tissue in the body.

E   the permanent teeth start to erupt at about 6 years of age.

96 Regarding the parotid gland:

A   the retromandibular vein passes through it.

B   the parotid duct opens onto the cheek opposite the second upper premolar tooth.

C   the parotid duct pierces the masseter muscle.

D   the mastoid process is a posterior relation.

E   an accessory parotid gland usually lies superficially on the masseter muscle.

97 Regarding normal development of the vertebral column:

A   fusion of the posterior aspects of the neural arches commences earliest in the cervical region.

B   fusion of the neural arches with the centrum commences earliest in the lumbar region.

C   five secondary ossification centres are present in each vertebra at puberty.

D   the dens may have more than one ossification centre.

E   the anterior margins of the thoracic vertebral bodies may appear irregular.

95 A **True** Each quadrant has two incisors, one canine, two premolars and three molars.

   B **True** Each quadrant has two incisors, one canine and two molars.

   C **False** The periodontal membrane is seen as a radiolucent line outlining the root. The lamina dura lies outside this, and appears as a radiopaque line around the root continuous with that of the adjacent teeth.

   D **True** It has a calcified inorganic content of 97%. Metallic fillings are more radiopaque than enamel.

   E **True** The permanent teeth in each quadrant erupt from medial to lateral. The lower teeth erupt 6–12 months earlier than the upper. Eruption is complete by about 20 years of age.

96 A **True** The retromandibular vein, the facial nerve and the external carotid artery all pass through the parotid gland.

   B **False** It opens onto the cheek opposite the second upper molar tooth.

   C **False** The parotid duct passes forwards over the masseter muscle, turns medially at its anterior border and pierces the buccinator.

   D **True** The parotid gland is related anteriorly to the angle of the mandible and the muscles attached to it. The external auditory meatus and temporomandibular joint lie superiorly. The styloid process lies medially, superficial to the carotid sheath.

   E **True** Several ducts open from an accessory gland into the main parotid duct.

97 A **False** Fusion of the neural arches posteriorly starts in the lumbar region at 1 to 2 years and proceeds cephalad to the cervical region up to 7 years of age. Fusion in the sacral region occurs last.

   B **False** Fusion of the neural arches with the centrum starts in the cervical region at 3 years and proceeds caudad to the lumbar region, which ossifies at 6 years of age. Fusion in the sacral region occurs last.

   C **True** These centres fuse at about 25 years.

   D **True** The dens may have two or three ossification centres; fractures may be simulated.

   E **True** There may be irregularity at the anterior and posterior margins of the thoracic vertebral bodies, representing vascular remnants and the basivertebral veins. The term Hahn's fissure relates to the anterior irregularity.

98   Regarding normal measurements in and around the spine:

A   in children the posterior laminar line of C2 may be up to 1 mm behind the posterior spinal line.

B   in children the atlanto-axial distance may be up to 8 mm.

C   the sagittal diameter of the cervical spinal canal at the level of C4 should not be less than 16 mm.

D   the prevertebral soft tissues in the adult should be less than 4 mm in width at the level of the nasopharynx.

E   the interpedicular distance should increase from L1 to L5.

99   Regarding the normal ligaments in the cervical spine:

A   the ligamenta flava are attached to the intervertebral discs and vertebral bodies anteriorly.

B   the membrana tectoria is a continuation of the posterior longitudinal ligament.

C   the ligamentum nuchae may calcify.

D   the cruciform ligament lies immediately behind the dens of the axis.

E   the apical ligament passes from the apex of the dens to the anterior edge of the foramen magnum.

100   In the vertebral canal:

A   the spinal cord usually ends at the level of the L1/2 disc space in adults.

B   the spinal cord has its maximum diameter at the level of C7.

C   the cauda equina is situated within the subarachnoid space.

D   the spinal cord is supported by the denticulate ligaments.

E   the artery of Adamkiewicz is the major arterial supply to the dorsolumbar spinal cord.

98 **A** **Truo** This physiological subluxation is caused by ligamentous laxity in children.

B **False** The atlanto-axial distance is less than 4–5 mm in children. It should measure no more than 3 mm in adults.

C **False** The sagittal diameter of the cervical spinal canal at the level of C4 may range from approximately 12–22 mm.

D **True**

E **True**

---

99 **A** **False** The ligamenta flava extend between adjacent laminae. The anterior longitudinal ligament is attached to the intervertebral discs and vertebral bodies anteriorly.

B **True** The posterior longitudinal ligament extends posterior to the vertebral bodies from the occipital bone to the sacrum. The membrana tectoria refers to that part which extends from the occipital bone to C2.

C **True** The ligamentum nuchae is part of the supraspinous ligament, which joins the tips of the spinous processes and extends from the external occipital protuberance to the sacrum.

D **True** The transverse part of the cruciform ligament passes between the lateral masses of the atlas and behind the dens to form the posterior part of the median atlanto-axial joint.

E **True**

---

100 **A** **True** 95% of cords end within the limits of the vertebral bodies of L1 and L2, 3% at the level of T12 and 2% at L3. At birth, the spinal cord usually ends at the L3 level.

B **False** The spinal cord has its maximum diameter at the level of C5.

C **True** The cauda equina consists of lumbar and sacral nerve roots and the filum terminale. As the segmental nerves leave the vertebral canal, they are invested in the meningeal covering of the cord.

D **True** The denticulate ligaments, layers of pia mater, lie laterally and are attached to the arachnoid and dura down to the level of the twelfth thoracic nerve.

E **True** It is an enlarged anterior radicular branch of a segmental artery in the T8–L4 region. It is left sided in about 60% of cases.

2 Techniques

1 **Regarding conventional high-osmolar contrast media:**
   A their viscosity at 20°C is approximately half that at 37°C.
   B the use of meglumine salts, as against sodium salts, is preferred for intravenous urography.
   C the incidence of severe adverse reactions to intra-arterial injections is about one third of those following intravenous injections.
   D their osmolality is five to eight times the physiological osmolality of plasma.
   E anaphylactoid reactions are usually dose-dependent.

2 **The following contrast medium agents are low-osmolar non-ionic monomers:**
   A meglumine ioglycamate (Biligram).
   B iothalamate (Conray).
   C iopamidol (Niopam).
   D meglumine and sodium ioxaglate (Hexabrix).
   E Iotrolan.

3 **The following should routinely receive low-osmolar contrast media (LOCM) rather than conventional high-osmolar contrast media (HOCM):**
   A patients with renal failure.
   B infants and the elderly.
   C poorly hydrated patients.
   D patients with myelomatosis.
   E patients with a strong history of allergy.

1 A **False**   Viscosity at 20°C is about twice that at 37°C.
   B **False**   Meglumine salts have a strong diuretic effect which
               therefore reduces the urinary iodine concentration in
               intravenous urography. The use of sodium salts is
               preferred.
   C **True**
   D **True**   The osmolality of low-osmolar contrast media is
               about one third the osmolality of conventional ionic
               contrast media, but still twice the physiological
               osmolality of plasma.
   E **False**   Anaphylactoid reactions are rarely dose-dependent.
               Hyperosmolar adverse reactions are dose-dependent.

2 A **False**   This is a low-osmolar bi-acidic dimer with an
               iodine:particle ratio of 6:3. It may be used for
               intravenous cholangiography.
   B **False**   This is a conventional high-osmolar ionic monomer
               with an iodine:particle ratio of 3:2.
   C **True**   A non-ionic monomer has an iodine:particle ratio of
               3:1.
   D **False**   This is a low-osmolar mono-acid dimer with an
               iodine:particle ratio of 6:2.
   E **False**   This is a low-osmolar non-ionic dimer with an
               iodine:particle ratio of 6:1.

3 A **True**
   B **True**   These groups are at increased risk of the adverse
   C **True**   hyperosmolar effects of contrast media.
   D **True**
   E **True**   And also those with a history of severe contrast
               medium reaction. Both groups are at increased risk
               of the anaphylactoid effect of contrast media.

4 Regarding contrast media:
A   the adverse reaction rate of intravenous low-osmolar contrast media is about one fifth that of intravenous conventional high-osmolar contrast media.
B   the urographic nephogram is produced by contrast medium in the renal arterioles.
C   physical or emotional stress increases a patient's susceptibility to an adverse reaction (following intravenous injection).
D   Gastrografin is indicated when attempting to demonstrate a tracheo-oesophageal fistula in an infant.
E   high-viscosity low-density barium should be used in double-contrast barium meal examinations.

5 Regarding the management of possible adverse reactions to intravenous contrast media:
A   intravenous metoclopramide should be given for nausea.
B   intravenous chlorpheniramine maleate (Piriton) is indicated in severe generalised urticaria.
C   intramuscular adrenaline 0.5–1 mg is a first-line drug to be used in the treatment of anaphylactoid shock.
D   corticosteroid prophylaxis is mandatory in asthmatic patients.
E   raising the patient's feet has no value in contrast-induced hypotension.

6 When using lignocaine as a local anaesthetic:
A   20 ml of a 1% solution is the maximum safe dose in adults.
B   it is effectively absorbed from mucous membranes.
C   convulsions are a recognised complication of toxicity.
D   there is an increased risk of lignocaine toxicity in patients on cimetidine.
E   it is contraindicated for use in acute porphyria.

4 A True   The quoted adverse reaction rate of conventional high-osmolar contrast media is about 5.8%.

 B False   The urographic nephrogram is produced by filtered contrast medium in the lumen of the tubules, mainly the proximal convoluted tubules.

 C True

 D False   Gastrografin is contraindicated because it is hyperosmolar and may cause pneumonitis and/or acute pulmonary oedema if aspirated. It may also cause dehydration by its hyperosmolar effect in the small intestine. Dilute barium or a low-osmolar non-ionic contrast medium should be used.

 E False   Low-viscosity high-density barium should be used.

---

5 A False   Confident reassurance alone is usually adequate. Intravenous antiemetics are rarely necessary.

 B True   This is an antihistamine. Intravenous corticosteroids should also be given.

 C True   Intravenous fluids, antihistamines, corticosteroids and nebulised beta-2-agonists may also be necessary. ECG monitoring, oximetry and blood pressure monitoring should also be carried out.

 D False   The value of corticosteroid prophylaxis remains unproven and controversial.

 E False   Simple manoeuvres alone may be effective in vasovagal syncope.

---

6 A True   The maximum safe dose of lignocaine for local anaesthesia is 200 mg.

 B True

 C True   Other side effects include agitation, euphoria, nausea, pallor, sweating and respiratory depression. Lignocaine toxicity can also cause hypotension, bradycardia and cardiac arrest.

 D True   Cimetidine inhibits the metabolism of lignocaine, thus increasing the risk of toxicity.

 E True   Lignocaine may induce acute porphyric crises. It is also contraindicated in hypovolaemia and complete heart block.

7   Regarding local anaesthesia in radiology:

   A paraesthesiae and sweating are early signs of lignocaine overdose.

   B adrenaline should always be added to lignocaine to prolong its local anaesthetic effect.

   C lignocaine is a constituent of Emla cream.

   D procaine is recommended in order to anaesthetise the pharynx prior to passage of the tube during enteroclysis.

   E respiratory depression as a result of lignocaine overdose may be reversed by naloxone.

8   Regarding pharmacological agents used in gastrointestinal radiology:

   A glucagon is a more potent smooth muscle relaxant than hyoscine butylbromide (Buscopan).

   B hyoscine butylbromide (Buscopan) may cause acute gastric dilatation.

   C glucagon is contraindicated in diabetic patients.

   D metoclopramide increases small bowel transit time.

   E with metoclopramide, extrapyramidal side effects are more likely to occur in children than in adults.

7 A True   In addition to pallor, speech disturbance, tremor and auditory hallucinations. These may progress to central nervous system and cardiovascular depression.

B False   Adrenaline, a vasoconstrictor, should not be added to lignocaine when used as a local anaesthetic in appendages or digits as it may produce ischaemic necrosis.

C True   Emla cream consists of a combination of lignocaine and another local anaesthetic agent. It is often used topically in children when it should be applied to the skin under an occlusive dressing 1–5 hours before any procedure.

D False   Procaine, a local anaesthetic, is poorly absorbed from mucous membranes. It is of no value as a surface anaesthetic. Lignocaine spray, which is well absorbed from mucous membranes, is used instead.

E False   Naloxone reverses respiratory depression caused by opioid analgesics. Respiratory depression caused by lignocaine overdose must be managed by supportive measures as there is no specific antagonist available.

---

8 A True

B True   A rare complication due to its anticholinergic action.

C False   Glucagon is contraindicated in patients with either a phaeochromocytoma or an insulinoma.

D False   Metoclopramide increases gastric peristalsis thus reducing small bowel transit time.

E True   Extrapyramidal side effects may occur if the dose exceeds 0.5 mg/kg.

9 **The following statements are true:**
   A intravenous glucagon is contraindicated in glaucoma.
   B intravenous glucagon is contraindicated in patients with phaeochromocytoma.
   C tachycardia is a recognised side effect of intravenous hyoscine butylbromide (Buscopan).
   D metoclopramide (Maxolon) decreases gastric emptying time.
   E metoclopramide (Maxolon) is contraindicated in patients with phaeochromocytoma.

10 **Regarding contrast media in the examination of the gastrointestinal tract:**
   A barium with a density of 250% w/v is ideal for a barium follow-through.
   B Gastrografin may be used in the treatment of meconium ileus.
   C barium may be used if aspiration is a possibility.
   D intraperitoneal barium has a mortality rate of approximately 50%.
   E a solution of 150 ml of Gastrografin in one litre of a flavoured drink is recommended to opacify the bowel prior to a CT examination.

9 A False   Intravenous Buscopan is contraindicated in
                closed-angle glaucoma due to its mydriatic action.
                Intravenous glucagon can be safely used as an
                alternative smooth muscle relaxant in this situation.
   B True   Glucagon administration in phaeochromocytoma
                may cause tumour release of catecholamines,
                resulting in sudden and marked hypertension. Other
                contraindications to glucagon are previous
                hypersensitivity reactions and known or suspected
                insulinoma.
   C True   Other anticholinergic side effects include blurring of
                vision, dry mouth and urinary retention.
   D True   This effect enhances the transit of barium during a
                follow-through examination.
   E True   Maxolon adminstration in phaeochromocytoma may
                induce an acute hypertensive response.

10 A False   Barium with a density of 250% w/v is suitable for a
                double-contrast barium meal, 100% w/v barium is
                recommended for a barium follow-through, and
                125% w/v is suitable for a barium enema.
   B True   The hypertonic Gastrografin draws water into the
                bowel, helping to dislodge the meconium. A
                diagnostic barium enema must be performed first.
   C True   When contrast media is likely to enter the lungs,
                either barium or a low-osmolar contrast medium
                should be used. Aspiration of Gastrografin causes
                pulmonary oedema.
   D True   Even with treatment, there is still a 50% mortality
                rate if barium leaks into the peritoneal cavity. If
                perforation is suspected, water-soluble contrast
                should be used.
   E False   A solution of 15 ml of Gastrografin in one litre is
                recommended. This dilution minimises artefacts
                arising from the contrast medium.

11   A barium swallow:
   A   provides better mucosal detail than does a Gastrografin swallow.
   B   should be performed with the patient prone when assessing oesophageal motility.
   C   is preferred to a Gastrografin swallow in suspected aspiration.
   D   requires high-density (250% w/v) barium when a single-contrast examination is carried out.
   E   should preferably be performed using a double-contrast technique when studying motility.

12   When performing a barium meal:
   A   the patient should be advised not to smoke on the day of the examination.
   B   complete large bowel obstruction is a contraindication.
   C   approximately 1000 ml of gas should be produced in the stomach for a satisfactory double contrast study.
   D   the RAO film demonstrates the lesser curve en face.
   E   the prone position should be adopted when attempting to demonstrate the anterior wall of the duodenum.

13   During a double-contrast barium meal examination:
   A   a supine patient position is optimal for demonstrating the fundus of the stomach.
   B   effervescent granules with good bubble formation should be used.
   C   the administration of hyoscine butylbromide (Buscopan) significantly affects the incidence of demonstrable gastro-oesophageal reflux.
   D   filling of the duodenal bulb with barium occurs more reliably with glucagon than hyoscine butylbromide (Buscopan).
   E   the areae gastricae are usually best seen on an erect film.

11 A True   Water soluble contrast media, such as Gastrografin,
                 give relatively poor mucosal detail.
    B True
    C True   Aspiration of Gastrografin causes a chemical
                 pneumonitis and acute pulmonary oedema; it is
                 therefore contraindicated in suspected aspiration.
                 Aspirated barium is usually coughed up without any
                 sequelae. Smaller volumes can be expectorated by
                 physiotherapy, but larger volumes can give rise to
                 severe respiratory embarrassment. Non-ionic contrast
                 media can be used safely in any situation where
                 there is likely to be aspiration or extravasation.
    D False   For a single-contrast study, a medium-density
                 (100% w/v), low-viscosity barium is indicated.
    E False   A single-contrast study is used when looking for
                 oesophageal dysmotility, compression or
                 displacement.

12 A True   Smoking causes increased gastric motility.
    B True
    C False   200–400 ml is an adequate volume of gas.
    D False   The RAO film demonstrates the antrum and greater
                 curve. The LAO film demonstrates the lesser curve
                 en face.
    E True

13 A False   It demonstrates the antrum and body of the stomach.
    B False   The ideal gas-producing agent should have no
                 bubble production, adequate gas production
                 (200–400 ml), non-interference with barium coating
                 and rapid dissolution with no residue. It should also
                 be cheap and easy to swallow.
    C False
    D False   Filling of the duodenal bulb with barium occurs more
                 reliably with Buscopan because it relaxes the pylorus.
    E False   They are best seen on the supine films.

14   For a small bowel barium follow-through examination:
A   the patient should be advised to empty their bladder prior to the examination.
B   Gastrografin added to the barium is recognised as a means of reducing small bowel transit time.
C   a suitable volume of barium to give a child is 15 ml/kg body weight.
D   serial supine abdominal radiographs should be taken after the barium has been ingested.
E   a pneumocolon technique is a recognised method of producing improved visualisation of the terminal ileum.

15   Regarding enteroclysis:
A   it is contraindicated in suspected small bowel obstruction.
B   to advance the catheter through the pylorus, it may be helpful to turn the patient onto their left side.
C   the catheter tip should ideally be positioned 5–10 cm beyond the ligament of Treitz.
D   barium should be infused at a rate of approximately 75 ml/min.
E   the procedure may be complicated by inducing a paralytic ileus.

16   Regarding a barium enema examination:
A   the procedure should not be performed within 4 weeks of a full thickness rectal biopsy.
B   toxic megacolon is an absolute contraindication.
C   a 15% w/v barium suspension is recommended for a single-contrast barium enema.
D   a Hampton's view (prone angled view of the sigmoid) is taken with the tube angled 30° cephalad.
E   perforation as a complication occurs in one in 1000 examinations.

14 **A** **False** A full bladder helps to raise the loops of small bowel out of the pelvis.

    B **True** Approximately 10 ml Gastrografin should be added to the barium in order to achieve this effect.

    C **False** In children, 3–4 ml/kg body weight is a suitable volume of barium.

    D **False** Prone films should be taken because the compression of the abdomen helps to separate the loops of small bowel.

    E **True** Reflux of air from the colon into the terminal ileum will aid visualisation in many patients.

15 **A** **False** Enteroclysis is not contraindicated in suspected small bowel obstruction. Barium will be diluted by the small intestinal fluid thus avoiding impaction.

    B **True** When on the left side, air collects in the antrum and duodenal bulb, and may encourage the tube to move towards the duodenum.

    C **True** If the tip of the tube is in the jejunum then the risk of reflux of barium into the stomach is minimised.

    D **True**

    E **True** Too fast an infusion of barium may distend and paralyse the jejunum, resulting in delayed filling of ileal loops.

16 **A** **False** In general a 7 day interval after a rectal biopsy allows the mucosa to grow over the biopsy site and thus minimises the risk of perforation.

    B **True** The friability of the colon in toxic megacolon renders it very susceptible to perforation.

    C **True** On the other hand a 125% w/v barium suspension is recommended for a double-contrast enema.

    D **False** The tube should be angled 30° caudally with the patient prone. This view helps to visualise the rectosigmoid.

    E **False** Perforation is the commonest serious complication of the barium enema. Its incidence is quoted at one in 12000.

17   With respect to a double-contrast barium enema examination:
   A   if to be performed within 3 days of a small bowel barium examination, the barium enema should be performed first.
   B   a patient with a prosthetic heart valve should be given antibiotic prophylaxis.
   C   the transverse colon is usually barium-filled in the supine position.
   D   ileal reflux of barium is minimised if air insufflation is performed with the patient supine.
   E   ileal reflux is increased when intravenous hyoscine butylbromide (Buscopan) is used.

18   Regarding examination of the gastrointestinal tract in children:
   A   barium investigation of a tracheo-oesophageal fistula should be performed with the patient supine.
   B   reduction of an intussusception should not be attempted radiologically if the symptoms have been present for over 24 hours.
   C   the explorator grid should be removed when screening infants under 1 year of age.
   D   when examining for gastro-oesophageal reflux the baby should be placed in the prone oblique position.
   E   for barium reduction of an intussusception the barium should be raised 100 cm above the table for 5 minutes, a maximum of three times.

19   With respect to sinogaphy:
   A   the catheter should be inserted to a maximum distance of 3 cm into the sinus track.
   B   water-soluble contrast medium should be used.
   C   A maximum of 20 ml of contrast medium should be injected.
   D   A radiopaque marker should be placed next to the opening of the sinus.
   E   Sinography performed during CT rarely demonstrates a more extensive track system than is visible on conventional fluoroscopy.

17 A False   The small bowel and stomach should be examined first as they will be clear of barium after a few hours, and the preparation for the enema will then remove the residual barium from the colon.

  B True   Transient bacteraemia may occur during a barium enema.

  C False   On a supine film the transverse colon is usually seen in good double-contrast. On a prone film the transverse colon is seen filled with barium as it is then dependent.

  D False   The ileocaecal valve is most commonly on the posteromedial wall of the caecum, and is therefore dependent in the supine position, making reflux of barium into the ileum likely.

  E True   Intravenous smooth muscle relaxants increase the likelihood of ileal reflux.

---

18 A False   The baby should be positioned prone to visualise contrast passing from the oesophagus into the trachea.

  B False   The contraindications to radiological reduction are the presence of peritonitis, perforation or advanced intestinal obstruction. Duration of the symptoms per se is not a contraindication.

  C True   By removing the grid, the radiation dose can be reduced by as much as 50%. Acceptable images will be obtained as there is little scatter.

  D True   Reflux is also best sought during episodes of crying.
  E True   If after this the intussusception has not reduced, it is considered radiologically irreducible.

---

19 A False   The catheter should be inserted as far as possible into the sinus track until resistance is felt. This should ensure optimum filling during injection.

  B True
  C False   The amount of contrast medium depends on the track system. If there is clinical evidence of a fistula, contrast should be injected until either reflux occurs or the fistula is shown.

  D True   This allows the orifice to be identified easily on all films, irrespective of the angle at which the film is taken.

  E False

20   Regarding biliary contrast media:
A   intravenous agents are actively excreted into the bile by hepatocytes.
B   they are concentrated in the normal gall bladder.
C   they bind to serum albumin.
D   an infusion technique for intravenous agents is preferable to bolus injection.
E   they are contraindicated in pregnancy.

21   Regarding oral cholecystography:
A   it may be useful in the diagnosis of acute cholecystitis.
B   the cystic duct and common bile duct are rarely visualised.
C   a fat-containing meal should be taken on the evening prior to the examination.
D   when a single dose technique is utilised, the cholecystographic agent should be taken approximately one hour before attempts are made to visualise the gall bladder.
E   tomography to show the gall bladder is usually necessary.

22   Regarding intravenous cholangiography:
A   visualisation of the biliary tree may be inadequate in up to approximately 45% of examinations in patients with normal hepatic function.
B   it is contraindicated in patients who have had a previous cholecystectomy.
C   if the contrast medium is infused too quickly, renal rather than biliary excretion may occur.
D   intravenous glucagon may improve visualisation of the common bile duct.
E   the mortality rate is approximately 1 in 5000 examinations.

20 A True   Oral agents are conjugated with glucuronic acid by hepatocytes to form conjugates which are more water-soluble.
   B True
   C True
   D True   Infusion of intravenous agents, rather than a bolus injection, results in an optimum plasma concentration with maximum biliary excretion and produces fewer side effects.
   E True   They are also contraindicated in combined hepatic and renal failure, and when there is a history of iodine hypersensitivity.

21 A False   Acute cholecystitis is a contraindication to oral cholecystography as the gall bladder will not opacify. Other contraindications include hepatorenal failure, dehydration, an IV cholangiogram within the previous week and previous cholecystectomy.
   B False
   C True   This empties the gall bladder and allows better subsequent filling.
   D False   The cholecystographic agent should be taken 14 hours prior to the appointment time. The control film must therefore be taken when the patient makes his/her appointment, as the gall bladder will already be opacified when the patient arrives for the investigation.
   E False   Tomography is often utilised in intravenous cholangiography.

22 A True
   B False   Intravenous cholangiography may provide useful information in post-cholecystectomy patients with recurrent symptoms of biliary tract disease.
   C True   An infusion of Biligram over 60 minutes (3–4 mg/kg/min) gives optimum plasma concentration with maximum biliary excretion. If it is infused too quickly, there is insufficient time for albumin binding, so renal excretion may occur.
   D True   It achieves this by three mechanisms: (1) contraction of the sphincter of Oddi, followed by relaxation; (2) increased choleresis and (3) increased hepatic blood flow.
   E True   Other complications include impairment of liver and renal function and the precipitation of abnormal paraproteins in patients with Waldenstrom's macroglobulinaemia.

23 **Regarding post-operative (T-tube) cholangiography:**
   A the examination should be performed at about the tenth day post-operatively.
   B a control film of the gall bladder area is required.
   C cholangiovenous reflux of contrast medium can occur.
   D retained calculi can be removed via the T-tube within a few days of post-operative cholangiography.
   E percutaneous extraction of retained biliary calculi may be complicated by pancreatitis.

24 **In endoscopic retrograde cholangiopancreatography (ERCP):**
   A the presence of a pancreatic pseudocyst is a contraindication to the procedure.
   B low-osmolar contrast medium with an iodine content of 150 mg/ml should be used to examine the pancreatic duct.
   C intravenous buscopan may allow easier identification of the ampulla of Vater.
   D if both the biliary tree and the pancreatic duct are to be opacified, the bile duct should be cannulated first.
   E hyperamylasaemia may occur in up to 70% of patients.

23 A True
    B True
    C True   The biliary ducts absorb contrast medium and
                  cholangiovenous reflux can occur with high injection
                  pressures.
    D False   When a calculus has been identified on the T-tube
                  cholangiogram, the patient should be discharged
                  with the T-tube clamped for at least 4 weeks to allow
                  the formation of a fistulous tract. The T-tube can then
                  be removed, and the stone extracted through the
                  fistulous tract with a basket.
    E True   Other complications of this technique include the
                  creation of false sinus passages, septicaemia and
                  vagal stimulation with shock.

24 A True   Other contraindications include acute pancreatitis,
                  severe cardiorespiratory disease, and any other
                  contraindication to endoscopy.
    B False   Dilute contrast medium (150 mg/ml) should be used
                  to examine the bile ducts to ensure calculi are not
                  obscured. A more concentrated contrast medium
                  (240 mg/ml) should be used for pancreatic duct
                  examination.
    C True   Due to its choloretic action.
    D False   The pancreatic duct should be cannulated first, and
                  the injection of contrast should be stopped as soon
                  as the lateral branches of the pancreatic duct are
                  seen.
    E True   Asymptomatic elevation of the serum amylase is
                  common and usually related to over-filling of the
                  pancreatic duct.

25 Regarding percutaneous transhepatic cholangiography (PTC):

A a platelet count of less than 100×10^9 l^{-1} is a contraindication to the procedure.

B a Chiba needle should be inserted through the liver via an anterior approach.

C the incidence of complications is primarily related to the number of passes prior to entering a duct.

D if contrast medium is seen in the intrahepatic lymphatics, the procedure should be terminated.

E internal biliary drainage is indicated if ductal calculi are demonstrated.

26 The following situations will increase the risk of bacteraemia during percutaneous transhepatic cholangiography (PTC):

A puncture of the portal venous radicles.

B overdistension of intrahepatic ducts.

C complete obstruction of the common bile duct.

D multiple percutaneous punctures.

E presence of cholangitis.

27 Regarding the use of contrast media in intravenous urography:

A the recommended dose in adults is 300 mg of iodine per kg of body weight.

B the recommended dose in children is approximately 1 ml of 370 contrast medium per kg of body weight.

C patients with renal failure require half the standard amount of iodine.

D the density of the nephrogram is determined by the degree of hydration of the patient.

E the density of the pyelogram is greater with sodium salts than with the equivalent meglumine salts for the same amount of injected iodine.

25 A **True**   Other contraindications include an elevated
              prothrombin time, hydatid disease and severe
              cardiopulmonary disease.
    B **False**   The Chiba needle (22G) is inserted in the mid-axillary
              line in the right seventh or eighth intercostal space. It
              is therefore inserted parallel to the plane of the table
              and advanced during suspended respiration through
              the right lobe of the liver.
    C **False**   The incidence of complications is not related to the
              number of passes. A maximum of 10–20 passes may
              be performed. The likelihood of success is directly
              related to the degree of duct dilatation and the
              number of passes made.
    D **False**   Excessive parenchymal injection may result in
              lymphatic opacification. This usually clears
              spontaneously and the procedure can be continued
              with the needle in a different position.
    E **False**   The presence of ductal calculi is a contraindication to
              endoprosthesis insertion.

26 A **True**
    B **True**
    C **True**   PTC should therefore be covered with prophylactic
    D **True**   antibiotics.
    E **True**

27 A **True**
    B **True**
    C **False**   Patients with renal failure require at least twice the
              standard amount of iodine (i.e. 600 mg iodine/kg).
    D **False**   Nephrogram density is determined by the contrast
              medium dose, the peak plasma contrast
              concentration and the glomerular filtration rate. It is
              independent of the degree of patient hydration.
    E **True**   Sodium salts produce less of an osmotic diuresis
              than meglumine salts because sodium is reabsorbed.
              Sodium salts therefore produce denser pyelograms.

28   For intravenous urography, low-osmolar contrast media are recommended in preference to high-osmolar media in patients with:

A   diabetes mellitus.
B   systemic lupus erythematosus.
C   sickle cell disease.
D   cardiac failure.
E   pulmonary emphysema.

29   Ureteric compression in intravenous urography:

A   is a recognised cause of vasovagal symptoms.
B   should be applied 15 minutes after the contrast medium has been injected.
C   is essential in neonates.
D   is acceptable even when there is an abdominal mass, provided that the mass is not tender.
E   is contraindicated if there has been recent abdominal surgery.

30   The following techniques are recognised as assisting radiographic visualisation on an IVU:

A   the tube should be angled 15° cephalad to obtain a coned post-micturition bladder view.
B   the ingestion of a fizzy drink to aid visualisation of the kidneys.
C   a prone film to aid ureteric visualisation.
D   35° anterior oblique renal views to improve delineation of the renal outline.
E   tomography centred on a point halfway between the table top and the anterior abdominal wall will aid visualisation of the renal outlines.

28 A True
    B False
    C True
    D True
    E False

29 A True   When this occurs the compression should be released, and the patient placed in the head down position.
    B False   If compression is indicated it should be applied 5 minutes post-injection.
    C False   Compression is not used in young infants.
    D False   The presence of an abdominal mass is an absolute contraindication to compression.
    E True   Other contraindications include renal trauma and renal obstruction.

30 A False   For a coned view of the bladder the tube is angled 15° caudad. It is centred 5 cm above the pubic symphysis.
    B True   In children a fizzy drink will produce a gas-filled stomach which acts as a window through which the kidneys can be seen.
    C True   When the patient is prone the ureters are more dependent aiding visualisation.
    D False   Oblique views of the kidney should be taken as 35° posterior obliques.
    E False   In general, the tomographic mid-point of the kidneys lies at one third the distance from the table top to the anterior abdominal wall at the inferior costal margin.

31 Regarding retrograde pyelography:

A   it is recognised as being useful in delineating a lesion inadequately shown on intravenous urography.

B   contrast medium with an iodine concentration of 340 mg/ml should be used.

C   50 ml of contrast medium is required to delineate the pelvicalyceal system.

D   in the presence of ureteric obstruction, contrast medium should be aspirated prior to withdrawal of the catheter.

E   pyelosinus backflow is usually asymptomatic.

32 Percutaneous renal puncture:

A   is recognised as being a useful technique in the evaluation of renal cysts.

B   is a fundamental part of the Whitaker Test.

C   should be directed towards the upper pole calyces for nephrostomy tube insertion.

D   may be complicated by an arteriovenous fistula in approximately 0.5% of cases.

E   is contraindicated in the presence of urinary tract infection.

33 Regarding micturating cystourethrography:

A   sedation should not be given.

B   water-soluble contrast medium with an iodine concentration of 100–150 mg/ml is recommended.

C   to demonstrate stress incontinence erect lateral views coned to the bladder only should be taken at rest, straining, and during micturition.

D   in male infants, the urethra should be imaged in the anterior oblique position.

E   lateral views should be taken when attempting to demonstrate vesicovaginal or rectovesical fistulae.

31 A True A retrograde examination is a useful adjunct to an inconclusive IVU to help demonstrate the site, length and lower limit of a lesion.

B False Dilute contrast medium (150–200 mg iodine/ml) should be used to ensure that small lesions are not obscured.

C False Usually 5–10 ml of contrast is needed to delineate the pelvicalyceal system. The injection should be terminated if the patient complains of loin pain.

D True This minimises the risk of development of a chemical pyelitis or a pyonephrosis.

E True Occasionally it may result in pain, fever and rigors.

---

32 A True If an apparently simple cyst is present together with unexplained fever, haematuria or pain, it may be helpful to drain the cyst via percutaneous renal puncture. Double contrast images of the cavity should then be obtained.

B True The Whitaker Test is used to distinguish between an obstructed and dilated system. A catheter is introduced percutaneously into the renal collecting system, and saline infused at a rate of 10 ml/min. A relative renal pelvis pressure (i.e. bladder pressure subtracted from renal pressure) less than 13 cm H_2O is normal.

C False The aim is to puncture a lower pole calyx, passing through the least depth of parenchyma to reach the collecting system. This reduces the chance of vascular damage.

D True

E False Percutaneous renal puncture and drainage via nephrostomy is not contraindicated in the presence of obstruction and infected urine; but prophylactic antibiotics should be given.

---

33 A False Young infants may need to be sedated particularly prior to catheterisation.

B True

C False These lateral views should include the sacrum and the symphysis pubis. These bony landmarks are used to assess bladder neck descent.

D True This ensures visualisation of the long axis of the urethra.

E True

34   Ascending urethrography:

A   is the examination of choice to demonstrate posterior urethral valves.

B   should not be performed within 2 weeks of urethral instrumentation.

C   requires about 20–40 ml water-soluble contrast medium.

D   is the radiographic examination of choice for demonstrating the prostatic urethra.

E   is complicated by intravasation of contrast medium in approximately 5% of cases.

35   Regarding hysterosalpingography (HSG):

A   it is contraindicated if there is a history of untreated salpingitis during the preceding 6 months.

B   it should be performed in the week preceding the menstrual period.

C   pethidine can be helpful if given as an analgesic before the procedure.

D   the procedure should be terminated if venous intravasation occurs.

E   pain may persist for up to 1–2 weeks after the procedure.

36   Regarding cavernosography:

A   it is a recognised procedure for investigating male erectile dysfunction.

B   a needle is positioned in each corpus cavernosum to ensure bilateral opacification.

C   approximately 20 ml of contrast medium is required to opacify the corpora cavernosa.

D   venous thrombosis is a recognised complication.

E   it is contraindicated in the presence of a proven urinary tract infection.

34 A False   Posterior urethral valves may not be demonstrated on this examination, as they only fill out and obstruct during micturition. Micturating cystourethrography is therefore the investigation of choice for suspected posterior urethral valves. The main indications for ascending urethrography are suspected urethral trauma and the assessment of a urethral stricture.

B True   This is due to the risk of intravasation of contrast medium from the mucosal damage that may have been caused by recent instrumentation.

C True

D False   The urethra is well seen as far as the membranous portion on ascending urethrography. To demonstrate the proximal prostatic urethra, a radiograph should be taken during micturition.

E True

---

35 A True   HSG is contraindicated until a course of antibiotics has been given and there is clinical evidence of successful treatment.

B False   HSG should be performed in the first week after the menstrual period.

C False   Pethidine stimulates smooth muscle contraction, which impedes the filling of the fallopian tubes with contrast medium.

D False   Venous intravasation may occur in approximately 4% of cases, but it is of little significance when water-soluble contrast media are used.

E True   It is postulated that this is due to pelvic irritation.

---

36 A True   Other indications are the demonstration of the extent of Peyronie's disease and the investigation of priapism and penile trauma.

B False   The corpora cavernosa on both sides are opacified from a unilateral contrast injection.

C True   20 ml of a low-osmolar contrast medium is recommended.

D True   Venous thrombosis can lead to priapism with impotence.

E False   The only contraindication is a history of hypersensitivity to contrast media.

37   In arthrography:
   A   control films are not usually recommended prior to the procedure.
   B   joint effusion is a contraindication because of the risk of introducing sepsis.
   C   negative contrast medium is absorbed from the joint within a few hours.
   D   delayed films may be useful in the investigation of a suspected loose body.
   E   adrenaline should not be added to the contrast medium.

38   Regarding shoulder arthrography:
   A   a single-contrast technique is usually recommended.
   B   the injection site lies at the same horizontal level as the coracoid process.
   C   the patient lies supine with the forearm pronated to allow easy needle entry into the joint space.
   D   CT examination requires a smaller volume of positive contrast medium.
   E   an axial radiograph is routinely performed following contrast injection.

39   In double-contrast knee arthrography:
   A   the needle is introduced at a point 1 cm posterior to the mid-point of the patella.
   B   about 15 ml of positive contrast medium is recommended.
   C   correct siting of the needle tip should be confirmed by aspiration of synovial fluid.
   D   the knee should be manipulated following contrast injection.
   E   any discomfort occuring in the joint at 12 hours is abnormal.

37 A False Control films should always be reviewed prior to the injection of contrast medium.

B False Joint effusion is not a contraindication to arthrography. The effusion should be aspirated prior to contrast injection in order to avoid dilution of contrast medium and bubble formation.

C False Negative contrast medium (air) may take up to 4 days to be completely absorbed from the joint space. Positive contrast medium is absorbed within a few hours.

D True

E False Adrenaline (0.1 ml of a 1:1000 solution) may be added to the contrast medium in order to delay its absorption from the joint space.

38 A False A double contrast study is usually performed using about 10 ml of positive contrast medium and 10 ml of air.

B False The injection site lies about 2 cm inferior and lateral to the tip of the coracoid process.

C False The patient lies supine with the forearm supinated and close to the body. This allows the long head of biceps to rotate away from the vertical path of the needle. In addition, the articular surface of the glenoid will face anteriorly avoiding damage to its labrum.

D True Up to 3 ml.

E True

39 A True Either via a medial or lateral approach into the patello-femoral joint space.

B False About 3 ml of positive contrast medium and 50 ml of air are injected.

C False Correct siting of the needle tip within the joint space is confirmed by a test injection of a small volume of contrast medium under fluoroscopic control. Contrast medium should flow rapidly around the joint.

D True This ensures even distribution of contrast medium within the joint.

E False Some discomfort may occur in the joint for up to about 2 days. The patient should be warned about this.

40 When performing myelography of the lumbar region:
   A a lumbar puncture within the preceding week is a contraindication.
   B approximately 10 ml of water-soluble contrast medium with an iodine strength of 240 mg/ml should be used.
   C contrast should be injected with the X-ray table tilted 15° head down.
   D routine frontal and lateral views of the lower thoracic cord are mandatory.
   E the patient should lie flat for 6 hours following the procedure.

41 In myelography:
   A lateral cervical puncture should be performed when there is a suspected mass lesion in the upper cervical canal.
   B less dilution of contrast medium occurs if the contrast flows cephalad in the spinal canal via a lumbar puncture than if the contrast flows caudad via a cervical puncture.
   C lateral cervical puncture is a recognised method of demonstrating the upper level of a spinal block.
   D a post-myelogram CT should be delayed for 24 hours after the myelogram in order to reduce the contrast density by dilution.
   E prolonged headache is a more frequent complication in females than in males.

42 In dacrocystography:
   A a macroradiography technique is recommended.
   B an occipitofrontal 20° control film is taken.
   C cannulation of the superior canaliculus is recommended.
   D 0.5–2.0 ml of Lipiodol ultrafluid is recommended.
   E bilateral rather than unilateral examination is common practice.

40 A True   A small amount of cerebrospinal fluid often leaks into the subdural or extradural space after a lumbar puncture, and if a second lumbar puncture is performed within a week of the first, the pool of leaked cerebrospinal fluid may be tapped instead of the subarachnoid space.

  B True
  C False   The table should be tilted 15° foot down during the injection to ensure pooling of contrast in the lumbar subarachnoid space.
  D True   In order to exclude unsuspected intraspinal tumours which can mimic a disc prolapse.
  E False   Following the procedure the patient should sit up so as to pool the contrast medium in the lumbosacral region. The patient is then allowed to remain ambulant if he/she wishes.

41 A False   This is a contraindication to direct cervical puncture. Other contraindications include cerebellar tonsillar herniation, suspected lumbar spinal dysraphism and certain spinal deformities leading to loss of the C1/2 interspace.

  B True
  C True
  D False   A delay is not needed between the myelogram and CT, unless the investigation is for syringomyelia, in which case a 24 hour delay is ideal to show the syrinx.
  E True   Post-myelographic headache occurs in 20–30% of patients, and about 10% will have more severe prolonged headaches, particularly females.

42 A True   Thus magnifying the image obtained.
  B False   The control film is an occipitomental film.
  C False   The lower canaliculus is usually cannulated preferentially as it is more convenient and functionally more important.
  D True
  E True   This enables comparison with the normal side, or, if abnormalities are bilateral (a common finding) the simultaneous demonstration of the two sides.

43 In sialography:

   A Lipiodol ultrafluid can be used as a contrast medium.

   B pain occurs more readily with a water-soluble contrast medium than with an oil-based agent.

   C a fine probe should be passed at least 2 cm into the parotid duct.

   D contrast medium should be injected into the parotid duct at a rate of approximately 2 ml/min.

   E an occlusal radiograph is useful in the evaluation of the parotid duct.

44 The following statements are true:

   A the anthropological baseline passes from the outer canthus of the eye to the centre of the external auditory meatus.

   B in a standard occipitofrontal projection the beam is angled cephalad.

   C in a submentovertical projection the radiographic baseline should be parallel to the film.

   D autotomography may be usefully employed in the lateral oblique view of the temporomandibular joint.

   E the coronoid process of the mandible is well shown on a standard occipitomental projection.

45 An appropriate radiographic centring point for:

   A a lateral view of the cervical spine is 2.5 cm posterior to the angle of the mandible.

   B an AP view of the shoulder is the acromion.

   C a frog lateral of the hips is the femoral head.

   D a PA chest radiograph is T4.

   E a PA view of the hand is the capitate.

43 A True   Either a water-soluble contrast medium or the
                    oil-based medium, Lipiodol, can be used in
                    sialography. Oil-based media are more viscous and, if
                    accidentally injected into the soft tissues, may remain
                    in situ for many years.
   B True
   C False   After passing the probe about 1 cm into the parotid
                    duct, resistance will be met where the duct
                    penetrates the buccinator muscle. The probe should
                    not be advanced any further.
   D False   Contrast medium should be injected very slowly at a
                    rate of approximately 0.2 ml/min.
   E False   This view is useful in evaluating the submandibular
                    duct.

44 A False   This is a description of the orbitomeatal (or
                    radiographic) baseline. The anthropological baseline
                    passes from the infraorbital point to the upper border
                    of the external auditory meatus. These two lines are
                    at an angle of about 10° to each other.
   B False   The beam is angled caudally and centred in the
                    midline above the external occipital protruberance to
                    emerge from the nasion.
   C True   The beam is directed at right angles to the
                    orbitomeatal plane and centred midway between the
                    external auditory meati.
   D False   Open and closed mouth views of the
                    temporomandibular joint do not employ patient
                    movement.
   E True

45 A True   This is approximately the level of C3.
   B False   For an AP view of the shoulder, the beam should be
                    centred on the coracoid process. For an axial view,
                    the centring point is the acromion.
   C False   A frog lateral view is taken of both hips
                    simultaneously. The hips are flexed, abducted and
                    laterally rotated, and the centring point is in the
                    midline, at the level of the femoral pulse.
   D True   For an AP chest radiograph the appropriate centring
                    point is the sternal notch.
   E False   For a PA view of the hand, the beam should be
                    centred on the head of the third metacarpal.

46 Regarding skull radiography:

A   the eye dose is up to 200 times greater with an AP projection than with a PA projection.

B   a horizontal beam lateral film is essential in the case of head injury.

C   in an occipito-frontal (OF) 20 film, the petrous ridges should be projected at or near the superior orbital margins.

D   a Towne's view requires 30° cranial angulation of the central ray.

E   for a submentovertical view, the radiographic baseline should be parallel with the film.

47 Regarding radiography of the facial bones and teeth:

A   the zygomatic arches are best demonstrated on the lateral view.

B   the central ray is angled 30° caudally for the standard occipitomental (OM) view.

C   when performing orthopantomography the patient should gently open and close their mouth during the exposure.

D   the maxillary antra are best shown on the occipitomental (OM) view.

E   the occlusal plane is a horizontal plane passing through the opposing biting surfaces of the teeth.

48 The following statements are true:

A   oblique views of the cervical spine are usually performed with the patient supine.

B   when taking an erect right anterior oblique view of the cervical spine the median sagittal plane of the head is parallel to the film.

C   in the AP oblique projection, the cervical intervertebral foraminae demonstrated are those on the side nearer the X-ray tube.

D   a right posterior oblique (RPO) view of the lumbar spine will demonstrate the left pars interarticularis.

E   for an oblique view of the lumbosacral junction, the patient is rotated approximately 45°.

46 A True   Therefore it is desirable to choose a PA projection
                     whenever possible.
    B True   To exclude air/fluid levels in the cranial cavity, the
                     ventricles or the sinuses.
    C False   On an OF 20 radiograph, the petrous ridges should
                     be projected onto the inferior orbital margins, leaving
                     an unobstructed view of the bony orbits.
    D False   A Towne's view is taken with the patient supine, the
                     tube angled 30° caudally and the beam centred on
                     the foramen magnum.
    E True   With the patient supine, the neck is fully
                     hyper-extended until the baseline is parallel to the
                     film. The beam should be centred midway between
                     the angles of the mandible.

47 A False   The zygomatic arches are visualised on
                     occipitomental projections, but an underpenetrated
                     SMV view gives the clearest demonstration. They
                     may also be seen on a Towne's view collimated to
                     include the zygomatic arches.
    B False   For a basic OM view the central ray is not angled.
                     For an OM 30 it is angled 30° caudally.
    C False   The patient should remain stationary. To prevent any
                     movement, most units utilise head clamps, a chin
                     rest and a bite rod.
    D True   Together with the frontal sinuses and anterior
                     ethmoids.
    E True

48 A False   These views are most commonly performed with the
                     patient erect.
    B True   The median sagittal plane of the trunk is about 45° to
                     the film.
    C True   In a PA oblique projection of the cervical spine, the
                     intervertebral foraminae that are seen are those
                     nearer the film.
    D False   Oblique views of the lumbar spine show the pars
                     interarticularis on the side to which the patient is
                     turned (e.g. RPO shows the right pars).
    E True

49 Regarding imaging of the breast:
  A compression should not be used during mammography when cysts are suspected.
  B ultrasound should be performed with a low frequency (3.5 MHz) transducer.
  C the standard mammography film series comprises a cranio-caudal view and a straight lateral view of each breast.
  D the nipple should be seen in profile in the standard mammographic views of the breast.
  E ductography involves the injection of 5 ml of a water-soluble contrast medium into a dilated duct.

50 Regarding lower limb lymphography:
  A the internal iliac lymph nodes are usually well demonstrated.
  B it should not be performed within 6 months of radiotherapy.
  C right-to-left crossover of lymphatics is more common than vice versa.
  D 7 ml Lipiodol ultrafluid should be used for each lower limb at an injection rate of 1 ml/min.
  E Hepatic oil embolism is a recognised complication.

51 In ascending venography of the lower limb:
  A a tourniquet applied above the ankle may occlude the normal anterior tibial vein.
  B the study is complete when the deep femoral vein has been demonstrated.
  C a single projection radiograph of the deep calf veins is adequate.
  D 60 ml iohexol 240 would be a suitable contrast medium.
  E at the end of the procedure the needle should always be flushed with normal saline.

49 A False

  B False   Ultrasound should be performed with a high frequency, high resolution transducer (5–10 MHz).

  C False   The standard series comprises a cranio-caudal and oblique lateral view of each breast.

  D True

  E False   0.5–1 ml of a water-soluble contrast medium should be injected into a duct slowly and the injection terminated when the patient experiences pain.

50 A False   The internal iliac, mesenteric, retrocrural, splenic and renal hilar nodes are not seen in this investigation.

  B False   Lymphography should not be performed within 3 weeks of radiotherapy as disruption of the lymph node architecture may allow oily contrast medium to pass into the systemic circulation.

  C True   Therefore visualisation of both sides is possible if only the right side is injected.

  D False   7 ml Lipiodol ultrafluid per lower limb should be injected over 45 minutes by a pump injector (approximately 0.2 ml/min).

  E True   This occurs when there is lymphatic obstruction and lymphaticoportal venous communication.

51 A True   The absence of anterior tibial vein filling by contrast is not therefore always indicative of venous thrombosis.

  B False   The deep femoral vein is only opacified in about 50% of cases when there is a loop connection with the superficial femoral vein, or when retrograde filling occurs during the Valsalva manoeuvre.

  C False   Radiographs of the deep calf veins should be obtained with the leg in internal and external rotation to avoid superimposition of bones and veins.

  D True

  E True   To avoid stasis of contrast medium in the leg leading to phlebitis.

52   In superior vena cavography:

A   contrast medium injection into a single median antecubital
vein is usually adequate.

B   the total volume of contrast medium injected should not
exceed 30 ml.

C   a Valsalva manoeuvre facilitates opacification.

D   catheterisation of both subclavian veins is rarely necessary to
obtain good opacification.

E   the normal azygos vein is often opacified.

53   Regarding portal venography:

A   indirect portal venography is performed via a transplenic
approach.

B   portal hypertension is a contraindication to the procedure.

C   for the transplenic approach, 50–60 ml of a low-osmolar
contrast medium (370 mg iodine/ml) should be injected at
8–10 ml/sec.

D   when using the transplenic approach, a larger volume of
contrast medium is required in patients with splenomegaly.

E   after transhepatic portal venography, a plug of gel-foam
should be placed in the catheter track.

54   Regarding intravenous digital subtraction angiography (IVDSA):

A   the basilic vein is preferred to the cephalic vein as a site of
access.

B   the right atrium is preferred to the superior vena cava as a
central site for the catheter tip.

C   abdominal compression may be useful when imaging
abdominal vessels.

D   contrast medium with a lower concentration of iodine per ml
than that used in intra-arterial DSA (IADSA) is recommended.

E   A 15 ml volume delivered centrally at a rate of 10 ml/sec is
suitable for each injection of contrast medium.

52 A False   Contrast medium should be injected into a vein in both arms simultaneously in order to opacify the superior vena cava.

B False   30 ml contrast medium should be injected into each arm.

C True

D True

E True

---

53 A False   Indirect portography results from injecting contrast into the coeliac or superior mesenteric arteries and obtaining delayed films of the portal vein.

B False   Portal venography is indicated to demonstrate the anatomy of the portal system in patients with portal hypertension. Direct percutaneous splenoportography can be used to measure portal venous pressure.

C True

D False   For transplenic portal venography, there is no need to increase the volume of contrast medium in splenomegaly. However, when performing indirect portography (i.e. late phase coeliac or superior mesenteric angiography) an increased volume of contrast is required in splenomegaly (about 70 ml low-osmolar contrast medium 370 mg iodine/ml at 8 ml/sec).

E True   This reduces the chance of blood or bile leakage into the peritoneum.

---

54 A True   It is more difficult to negotiate a catheter through the cephalic vein in the region of the clavipectoral fascia.

B True   The right atrium is the optimal site for contrast injection as it produces good mixing of blood from the superior and inferior vena cavae.

C True   Subtraction errors due to bowel gas movement may be reduced by abdominal compression and intravenous Buscopan.

D False   IVDSA uses full-strength contrast medium (about 350 mg iodine/ml). IADSA uses contrast medium diluted to about one-third to one-half of the normal concentration.

E False   A 35 ml volume delivered at a rate of 20 ml/second is suitable.

55 Regarding angiographic equipment:

A the French size of a catheter is a measure of the circumference of the catheter tip.

B polyethylene catheters are stiffer than polyurethane catheters and this provides better torque control.

C guide wires consist of two inner straight wires with an outer wire coiled around them.

D a typical guide wire measures 0.035 inches (0.89 mm) or 0.038 inches (0.97 mm) in diameter.

E a typical catheter measures 60–100 cm in length.

56 Regarding angiography:

A the hole in the vessel wall produced by a 6 French catheter has an area four times larger than that of a 3 French catheter.

B sheaths are sized according to the largest size catheter that they will accommodate.

C single-wall arterial puncture requires a two-part needle.

D the catheter tip should be positioned about 5–10 cm above the aortic bifurcation in lumbar aortography.

E the most reliable guide to the position of the common femoral artery for percutaneous puncture is the site of maximal pulsation.

57 A low-osmolar contrast medium with an iodine concentration of 350 mg/ml delivered at these injection volumes and rates would be appropriate for use in the following conventional arteriographic examinations:

A lumbar aortography: approximately 50 ml volume; rate 8–12 ml/sec.

B superior mesenteric arteriography: approximately 50 ml volume; rate 6–10 ml/sec.

C pulmonary arteriography: approximately 20 ml volume; rate 8–10 ml/sec.

D right coronary arteriography: approximately 15 ml volume; rate 10 ml/sec.

E common carotid arteriography: approximately 12 ml volume; hand injection.

55 A True
  B False   Polyurethane catheters are stiffer than polyethylene catheters.
  C True   One inner straight wire runs the whole length of the guide wire to reduce the risk of fracturing. The other inner wire terminates near the end of the guide wire to produce a soft flexible tip; it may be movable for variable stiffness of the tip.
  D True   Typical length of a guide wire is 100–150 cm.
  E True   Most diagnostic angiography is performed with 4 French or 5 French catheters.

56 A True   A 3 French catheter produces a hole 1 mm in diameter. A 6 French catheter produces a hole 2 mm in diameter. This represents a four fold increase in area ($\pi \times$ radius^2).
  B True
  C False   Double-wall arterial puncture requires a two-part needle, which consists of a bevelled central stilette and an outer blunt cannula. Single-wall arterial puncture uses a one-part needle with a central bore.
  D True   This site lies at the level of L3/4.
  E True

57 A True
  B True   Approximately the same volume and rate of contrast medium injection for coeliac arteriography. Inferior mesenteric arteriography requires about 15 ml volume at rate 3–5 ml/sec.
  C False   Pulmonary arteriography requires 40–50 ml volume at rate 20–25 ml/sec.
  D False   Right coronary arteriography requires 3–8 ml volume by hand injection. Left coronary arteriography requires 5–10 ml volume by hand injection.
  E False   A contrast medium iodine concentration of 350 mg/ml is too high for common carotid arteriography. About 12 ml low-osmolar contrast medium with an iodine concentration of not more than 300 mg/ml is suitable. This should be given by hand injection.

58   In pulmonary angiography:

   A   the catheter tip should be sited at the bifurcation of the pulmonary artery.

   B   anteroposterior and lateral projections should be obtained routinely.

   C   pigtail catheters are not suitable due to risk of rupture of the right ventricular chordae tendinae on withdrawal.

   D   films which record the arterial, capillary and venous phases should be obtained.

   E   pulmonary hypertension is a contraindication.

59   In angiocardiography:

   A   the right side of the heart is studied via a catheter passed retrogradely from the femoral artery.

   B   a cine-film frequency of 15 frames per second is usually adequate.

   C   a pigtail catheter is suitable for left ventricular injections.

   D   the right anterior oblique projection will demonstrate the mitral valve satisfactorily.

   E   a rise in the incidence of ectopic beats occurs with increasing contrast injection rates.

60   In coronary arteriography:

   A   the Sones technique requires right and left coronary artery catheters.

   B   the tip of the left Judkins' coronary artery catheter is more curved than that of the right.

   C   a 40° caudal-cranial view is ideal for visualisation of the left main-stem coronary artery.

   D   coronary arteriography is usually preceded by left ventricular angiography.

   E   coronary artery dissection is not usually clinically significant.

58 A False The catheter tip should be sited 1–3 cm above the pulmonary valve, i.e. below the bifurcation of the pulmonary artery.
 B False The anteroposterior projection is adequate. Oblique views may also be useful. A lateral projection is of no value in a main-stem pulmonary artery injection due to superimposition.
 C False Pigtail catheters are most commonly used. Insertion of the guidewire to straighten out the end of the catheter, prior to withdrawal, avoids this complication.
 D True
 E False Pulmonary hypertension is an indication for pulmonary arteriography. However, there is increased risk that the procedure may be complicated by cardiorespiratory failure in these circumstances.

59 A False The right heart is studied via a catheter passed anterogradely into a peripheral vein. In adults, the left heart is studied via a catheter passed retrogradely from the femoral artery. In children, it is usually possible to manipulate a venous catheter through a patent foramen ovale to examine the left heart.
 B False About 25–80 frames per second are required.
 C True
 D True
 E True

60 A False The Sones technique uses a single catheter via a brachial arteriotomy.
 B True To aid engagement of the coronary ostia by the catheters.
 C True
 D True Left ventricular angiography is carried out using a right anterior oblique projection.
 E False Coronary artery dissection is usually followed by cardiac arrest.

61   Recognised complications of diagnostic angiography include:

A   retroperitoneal haemorrhage following transfemoral puncture.
B   brachial plexus injury.
C   arteriovenous fistula formation.
D   cholesterol embolisation.
E   bacterial endocarditis.

62   The following statements are true of vascular interventional techniques:

A   prior to balloon dilatation of a leg vessel, the guidewire must be removed.
B   iliac arteries are preferably dilated antegradely from a femoral puncture on the side opposite the lesion.
C   heparin should not be given during angioplasty due to the increased risk of haematoma formation.
D   following an embolisation procedure, the patient may have a fever for up to 10 days.
E   embolic material should always be radiopaque.

63   The ideal radiopharmaceutical should:

A   have a half-life that is approximately four times the length of the scintigraphic examination.
B   emit mainly charged particle emissions.
C   produce emissions with an energy between 80 keV and 300 keV.
D   localise only in the area of interest.
E   be mono-energetic.

61 A True   Transfemoral puncture may also be complicated by haematoma formation in the femoral sheath, subperitoneal and intraperitoneal spaces, scrotum and fascial planes of the thigh.

   B True   This may complicate axillary artery puncture. It occurs either due to primary nerve injury or secondary to extrinsic compression of the brachial plexus by haematoma.

   C True   Other complications local to the puncture site include arterial thrombus and spasm, subintimal dissection, sepsis, false aneurysm and perivascular extravasation of contrast medium.

   D True
   E True   Other complications remote from the puncture site include subintimal dissection, arterial thrombosis and spasm, embolisation, catheter knotting, guide wire fracture and septicaemia.

---

62 A False   Dilatation should be performed with the guidewire remaining across the stenosis/occlusion until the procedure is completed.

   B False   Iliac arteries are preferably dilated retrogradely via an ipsilateral puncture.

   C False   The patient should be anticoagulated during an angioplasty procedure using 3000–5000 units of heparin.

   D True   Post-embolisation syndrome comprises fever, pain, leucocytosis and a general feeling of being unwell. It should only be diagnosed when other treatable causes of the patient's condition (e.g. infection) have been excluded.

   E False   Non-opaque emboli should always be injected as a suspension in contrast medium so that they are visible as filling defects during the injection sequence.

---

63 A False   The half-life should be of a similar length to the duration of the examination.

   B False   The radionuclide should emit gamma rays and there should be no charged particle emissions (i.e. alpha and beta emissions) as these increase radiation dose without contributing to image quality.

   C True   This ensures that the emissions penetrate tissue, but will be stopped by the detector.

   D True
   E True

64   Regarding isotope brain scanning:
A ^{99m}Tc HMPAO does not cross the blood-brain barrier.
B ^{99m}Tc diethylene triamine pentaacetic acid (DTPA) is useful in clinical practice.
C   when using ^{99m}Tc pertechnetate, perchlorate must be given beforehand.
D   imaging should be commenced 1–2 hours following injection.
E   single photon emission computed tomography (SPECT) is mandatory when ^{99m}Tc HMPAO is used.

65   Regarding isotope bone scanning:
A   it is a highly specific investigation.
B ^{99m}Tc methylene diphosphonate (MDP) remains stable for 48 hours.
C   20% of the injected ^{99m}Tc MDP localises in bone.
D   to ensure adequate counts the patient should not pass urine between the isotope injection and imaging the static phase.
E   the blood pool phase should be imaged approximately 15 minutes after injection.

64 A False ^{99m}Tc HMPAO is a lipophilic radiopharmaceutical which does cross the blood-brain barrier.

    B True   The three principal radiopharmaceuticals used for brain imaging are ^{99m}Tc DTPA, ^{99m}Tc pertechnetate and ^{99m}Tc glucoheptonate.

    C True   Pertechnetate is the cheapest of the three radiopharmaceuticals, but has the disadvantage that it is the only one to accumulate in the choroid plexus, thyroid and salivary glands. This is prevented by the administration of perchlorate 30–45 minutes before the investigation.

    D False   The dynamic phase is imaged immediately following the injection of isotope, and the static images are taken 1–2 hours post injection.

    E True   Anatomical detail is better displayed using SPECT at any time from 2 minutes to 8 hours after injection.

65 A False   The bone scan is highly sensitive but non-specific as any lesion in bone (e.g. fracture, infection, tumour or healing bone) will show as an area of increased activity.

    B False   Preparation involves reduction of the pertechnetate ion. After 6 hours this may reoxidise back to free pertechnetate which would localise in the thyroid and the stomach and thus degrade the scan.

    C True   The remainder is excreted by the kidneys.

    D False   The patient should be encouraged to drink plenty of fluid and to empty the bladder regularly so as to reduce the radiation dose to the bladder.

    E False   The blood pool phase should be imaged 1 to 2 minutes post injection. The blood flow phase and the static phase should be imaged in the first 30 seconds and at 3–4 hours respectively.

66 Regarding isotope examinations of the thyroid and parathyroid glands:

  A ^{131}I is the most frequently used agent for examination of the thyroid.

  B ^{123}I has a half-life of 13 hours.

  C prior use of an intravenous non-ionic contrast medium will result in poor uptake of the isotope within the thyroid gland.

  D the thyroid images should be obtained with a converging collimator.

  E the parathyroids are imaged via a subtraction technique, subtracting the ^{201}Tl image from the ^{99m}Tc image.

67 Regarding the radiopharmaceuticals used for lung ventilation studies:

  A when using ^{133}Xe a single breath technique is employed.

  B when using ^{127}Xe, the ventilation study must be performed prior to the perfusion study.

  C a krypton ventilation study can be performed simultaneously with the perfusion study.

  D when using krypton, lateral oblique views should be avoided because of the confusion caused by overlap of the two lungs.

  E ideally, ^{99m}Tc DTPA aerosols should not be used in patients with chronic airways disease.

66 A False ^{131}I is used mainly in the study of metastatic thyroid cancer. It is not used for routine thyroid imaging due to the high radiation dose from beta-emission. The most frequently used agents are ^{123}I and ^{99m}Tc pertechnetate.

B True ^{131}I has a half-life of 8 days.

C True Uptake of either ^{99m}Tc pertechnetate or iodine is inhibited by recent high ingestion of iodine.

D True This gives high resolution images. Note that this is at the expense of increased imaging time and some degree of image distortion.

E False ^{201}Tl is taken up by the thyroid and parathyroid glands. ^{99m}Tc is taken up by the thyroid gland only. Parathyroid images are therefore obtained by subtracting the ^{99m}Tc image from the ^{201}Tl image.

---

67 A True Because of the high radiation dose, a single breath technique is employed. Images are taken in one position only (usually posterior). The images obtained are in inspiration, equilibrium and in two washout phases.

B False When using ^{133}Xe, the ventilation study must be performed first otherwise image quality would be compromised by scattered radiation from the higher energy ^{99m}Tc gamma rays used for the perfusion scan. ^{127}Xe emits gamma rays with higher energy than ^{133}Xe and ^{99m}Tc and so can be used to perform a ventilation study after a perfusion scan.

C True If dual energy data acquisition is performed; as krypton emits gamma rays with an energy of 190 keV and ^{99m}Tc emits gamma rays with an energy of 140 keV.

D False In a krypton ventilation study, six views of the lungs should be obtained: anterior; posterior; RPO; LPO; right lateral; and left lateral.

E True Aerosols clump and therefore cause focal areas of increased uptake in patients with chronic airways disease.

68   Regarding perfusion isotope lung imaging:

A   it should be performed after a ventilation scan in order to diagnose pulmonary embolism.

B   the patient should be imaged in the supine position to maximise visualisation of the lung apices.

C   the ^{99m}Tc-macroaggregated albumin particles occlude less than 0.5% of the total capillary bed of the lung.

D   the syringe should not be shaken before the injection as this may damage the albumin macroaggregates.

E   respiratory failure may be induced in patients with pulmonary hypertension.

69   Regarding isotope examinations of the urinary tract:

A ^{99m}Tc DMSA has specific affinity for the proximal convoluted tubular tissue.

B ^{99m}Tc DTPA is excreted by glomerular filtration.

C ^{99m}Tc DMSA is never used to obtain a renogram curve.

D   the peak of the renogram should occur at 3–5 minutes.

E ^{99m}Tc MAG-3 is excreted by glomerular filtration.

68 A False   A normal perfusion scan will exclude a diagnosis of pulmonary embolism. A perfusion scan should therefore be performed first, and the ventilation scan only needs to be done if the perfusion scan is abnormal.

B False   Imaging should be performed in the sitting position. The injection should be given with the patient supine.

C True   The bronchial circulation maintains pulmonary nutrition so there is no irreversible tissue damage.

D False   The syringe should be shaken so as to prevent particles settling, as this would cause clumping on the image.

E True   A slow injection should be given in patients with pulmonary hypertension, and microspheres should be used whenever possible. Perfusion scanning is contraindicated in patients with right to left cardiac shunts due to the possibility of systemic microemboli.

69 A True ^{99m}Tc DMSA is bound to plasma proteins and is cleared from the blood by renal tubular absorption.

B True   When injected intravenously, ^{99m}Tc DTPA is distributed throughout the extracelluar space. It is excreted rapidly from the body by glomerular filtration.

C True ^{99m}Tc DMSA is used only for static renal imaging. ^{99m}Tc MAG-3 and ^{99m}Tc DTPA are the commonest radiopharmaceuticals used to obtain a renogram.

D True   The normal renogram comprises three phases: the vascular phase, the secretory phase and the excretory phase. The peak of the renogram occurs at 3–5 minutes post injection, and it takes 10–15 minutes for the activity to drop to half its peak value (the clearance half-time).

E False ^{99m}Tc MAG-3 is excreted by tubular secretion and has an extraction efficiency three times greater than ^{99m}Tc DTPA.

70   Regarding radionuclide investigation of the gastrointestinal tract:

A   patient preparation is not required for a radionuclide Meckel's diverticulum scan.

B   gastrointestinal bleeding will only be detected if the rate of blood loss is greater than approximately 0.5 ml/min.

C   a recent barium study may mask a bleeding site.

D   gastro-oesophageal reflux may be demonstrated with ^{99m}Tc sulphur colloid.

E   a full bladder is encouraged in a Meckel's scan in order to elevate and separate small bowel loops.

71   Regarding cardiovascular radionuclide imaging investigations:

A   red cells are labelled with chromium ions.

B   multiple gated acquisition (MUGA) may not be possible if the patient is in atrial fibrillation.

C ^{201}Tl is taken up by skeletal muscle.

D   methoxy isobutyl isonitrile (MIBI) is excreted via the hepatobiliary route.

E   in myocardial infarct imaging with ^{99m}Tc pyrophosphate, infarcts show tracer uptake from 24 hours and do so for up to 10 days.

70 A False   Nil by mouth for 6 hours unless it is an emergency. Prior administration of an H_2 blocker or pentagastrin is also advised so as to enhance detection by increasing the uptake of ^{99m}Tc pertechnetate into gastric mucosa and inhibiting its release into the lumen of the stomach or bowel.

   B True

   C True   Barium causes significant attenuation of gamma photons and may mask a bleeding site.

   D True   In adults, orange juice labelled with ^{99m}Tc colloid may be used to demonstrate reflux, and in young children a normal milk feed may be similarly labelled.

   E False   The bladder should be empty. A full bladder may obscure the Meckel's diverticulum.

---

71 A False   Red cells are labelled with ^{99m}Tc pertechnetate, but before this they are primed with an injection of stannous ions. The stannous ions reduce the pertechnetate and allow it to bind to the red blood cells.

   B True   If the patient has an arthythmia, the computer cannot identify an acquisition cycle.

   C True   Distribution of thallium is related to blood flow and metabolism. It is mainly taken up by muscle and thyroid, but some uptake occurs in the liver, spleen and kidney. It is used for myocardial perfusion imaging.

   D True   The gall bladder may therefore appear as an area of increased tracer uptake on a ^{99m}Tc MIBI scan. A drink of milk or a fatty meal 30–60 minutes after injection helps to clear the radiopharmaceutical from the liver and gall bladder so that myocardial perfusion can be imaged.

   E True   The size and intensity of myocardial uptake is related to infarct size.

72   The following statements are correct:

A   In ^{67}Ga scintigraphy uptake within the bowel is often a normal feature.

B ^{99m}Tc tin colloid is taken up in the liver by the hepatocytes.

C   In colloid scintigraphy, focal liver disease may be mimicked by overlying breast tissue.

D   In normal cholescintigraphy, the gall bladder should be visualised by 1 hour.

E   Tricyclic antidepressants should be stopped prior to a radioiodine M-iodobenzylguanidine (MIBG) scan for phaeochromocytoma.

73   In ultrasound of the upper abdomen:

A   the spiral valve of the cystic duct will frequently produce an acoustic shadow.

B   assessment of gall bladder wall thickness is preferably carried out after a fatty meal.

C   reflectivity of the normal liver parenchyma is slightly higher than that of the normal renal cortex.

D   an intercostal approach is optimal for examining the adrenal glands.

E   hepatic veins have highly reflective walls.

72 A **True**   Bowel activity is prominent up to 72 hours and is one
of the main drawbacks of ^{67}Ga imaging for
abdominal infection. Delayed imaging is essential.

   B **False**   Radiolabelled colloids are taken up by the Kupffer
cells in the liver.

   C **True**   There is considerable variation in normal liver
appearances. For example, focal abnormalities can
also be mimicked by rib impressions, hepatic veins,
and the impression of the right kidney.

   D **True** ^{99m}Tc N-substituted iminodiacetic acid (HIDA) is taken
up by hepatocytes and secreted into the bile in the
same way as is bilirubin. By one hour the gall
bladder is normally visualised.

   E **True**   Tricyclic antidepressants block MIBG uptake, as does
reserpine, labetalol and cocaine. The thyroid should
be blocked before MIBG scanning with potassium
perchlorate or Lugol's iodine.

73 A **True**   This should not be mistaken for a stone in the cystic
duct.

   B **False**   The normal gall bladder is contracted and
thick-walled after a fatty meal. These appearances
cannot be distinguished from pathological
contraction. Therefore, gall bladder wall
measurements should only be carried out in the
fasting state, when wall thickness is normally less
than 3 mm.

   C **True**   Reflectivity of the normal liver parenchyma is also
slightly higher than that of the spleen.

   D **True**
   E **False**   Hepatic veins have poorly reflective walls. Portal
veins have highly reflective walls.

74   In ultrasound of the pancreas:
   A   the pancreatic duct cannot normally be visualised.
   B   an oral fluid load may be helpful.
   C   the pancreas is more frequently visualised with the patient erect than in any other position.
   D   the normal pancreas is homogeneous with a reflectivity greater than or equal to that of the liver.
   E   the maximum anteroposterior (AP) diameter of the normal pancreatic head is 15 mm.

75   Regarding urinary tract ultrasound:
   A   the renal sinus is normally echogenic.
   B   renal lengths are preferably measured in the anteroposterior plane for standardisation.
   C   maternal collecting system dilatation does not normally occur before the third trimester of pregnancy.
   D   the full bladder appears rectangular-shaped in transverse section.
   E   a jet of urine entering the bladder is commonly observed.

76   In ultrasound scanning of the testes:
   A   a 3.5 MHz transducer frequency is recommended.
   B   a water bath is not useful.
   C   the normal testis is heterogeneous in texture.
   D   the mediastinum testis is seen as a thin reflective band lying longitudinally.
   E   the head of the epididymis is of similar reflectivity to the testicular tissue.

74 A False   The pancreatic duct can normally be visualised in almost 90% of patients. Its maximum diameter, in the region of the pancreatic body, is up to 2 mm in patients under 60 years of age. The calibre of the pancreatic duct increases with age.

B True   This produces an acoustic window through the stomach. This helps to visualise the pancreatic body and tail when the patient is turned onto their left side, and the pancreatic head and uncinate process when the patient is turned onto their right side.

C True

D True   Variations in the level of reflectivity of the pancreas probably relate to the degree of fat content; this commonly increases after 60 years of age.

E False   The maximum AP diameter of the pancreatic head is 25 mm. The pancreatic body has a maximum AP diameter of 15 mm.

75 A True   Due to fat surrounding the renal collecting system and blood vessels. This reflectivity is reduced in neonates.

B False   Renal lengths are measured by rotating the probe around the long axis of the kidney and recording its longest length.

C False   Mild collecting system dilatation occurs as early as 12 weeks gestation. This increases throughout pregnancy until term, when dilatation is usually more marked on the right side. Following delivery, the dilatation decreases but may persist for at least 3 months.

D True

E True   Due to the effect of normal ureteric peristalsis.

76 A False   A high resolution transducer in the frequency range 7.5–10 MHz is desirable.

B False   A water bath clears the organ being examined from near field interference and ensures that the organ lies within the focal zone of the transducer.

C False   The normal testis is acoustically homogeneous. It is of medium reflectivity.

D True   It is a normal structure representing condensations of connective tissue within the testicular stroma.

E True   But the rest of the epididymis is less reflective than testicular tissue.

77   A 7.5 MHz frequency transducer is suitable for scanning the:
A   orbit.
B   thyroid.
C   salivary glands.
D   breast.
E   neonatal hip.

78   In normal neonatal ultrasound:
A   the pancreas is markedly echogenic.
B   the neonatal adrenal gland is more easily visualised than that of the adult.
C   the renal pyramids appear prominent.
D   a 3.5 MHz linear array transducer is preferred when scanning the brain.
E   the tri-radiate cartilage cannot be identified.

79   In ultrasound of the neonatal brain:
A   the anterior fontanelle is preferentially used as a window for scanning.
B   the choroid plexus is highly echogenic.
C   the corpus callosum is echopoor.
D   the cavum septum pellucidum can be visualised in about 95% of full-term infants.
E   a 7.5 MHz linear array transducer is ideal.

77 A True
    B True
    C True
    D True
    E True

78 A False   The pancreas is echopoor in neonates.
    B True   For several reasons: the neonatal adrenal gland is
                proportionally larger; there is less neonatal perirenal
                fat; and higher frequency transducers are used,
                improving resolution. The normal adrenal cortex
                appears echopoor and the medulla echogenic.
    C True   The renal pyramids are large and echopoor
                compared with the thin echogenic cortex. These
                neonatal appearances alter between 2 and 6 months
                of age when the adult pattern emerges.
    D False   A 5–7.5 MHz sector transducer should be used.
    E False   The tri-radiate cartilage is seen as an echopoor area
                between the bony ilium and ischium. Ultrasound of
                the neonatal hip is successfully carried out using the
                cartilaginous femoral head as an acoustic window
                into the acetabulum.

79 A True   The posterior fontanelle and temporo-parietal bone
                can also be used.
    B True
    C True
    D False   The cavum septum pellucidum can be visualised in
                about 50% of all full-term infants. By 6 months of
                age, its incidence is similar to that reported in adults
                (15–20%).
    E False   This technique requires a sector transducer. A linear
                array transducer has a long rectangular scan head
                and a field of view which is unsuitable for
                visualisation of the whole brain through a small
                acoustic window.

80 In endoscopic ultrasound examination of the oesophagus:
A patient preparation should include drinking at least 1 l of fluid.
B the heart valves can be identified.
C manometry is carried out as part of the procedure.
D pH monitoring is part of the procedure.
E all the layers of the oesophageal wall can be identified.

81 In transrectal prostatic ultrasound:
A the reflective peripheral zone constitutes the major part of the normal gland.
B patients are examined prone.
C an anal stricture is a contraindication.
D no bowel preparation is required.
E the seminal vesicles are highly echogenic.

82 Regarding interventional techniques in ultrasound:
A the transducer should be sterilised by autoclaving following ultrasound guided puncture and biopsy.
B needle position within the tissues is demonstrated by the highly echogenic needle shaft.
C fine-needle biopsy is safely performed on an outpatient basis.
D local anaesthesia is necessary prior to transrectal guided biopsy of the prostate gland.
E prophylactic intravenous antibiotics are recommended prior to transrectal guided biopsy of the prostate gland.

80 A **False**   The ultrasound probe is attached to a rubber bag
                    containing water so that acoustic contact can be
                    maintained between the oesophageal wall and probe.
    B **True**   Identification of the heart valves helps to define local
                    anatomy.
    C **False**   Endoscopic ultrasound defines anatomy rather than
                    function. Manometry requires a perfused multilumen
                    tube.
    D **False**   pH monitoring requires a pH probe to be positioned
                    in the lower oesophagus for 24-hour monitoring.
    E **True**

81 A **True**   The peripheral zone constitutes 70% of the normal
                    gland. It is more reflective than the remaining
                    transitional and central zones of the gland.
    B **False**   Patients are examined in the left lateral position.
    C **True**
    D **True**
    E **False**   The seminal vesicles are echopoor with fine internal
                    echoes.

82 A **False**   Ultrasound transducers do not tolerate autoclaving.
                    Sterility is achieved by the use of sterile rubber
                    coverings for the transducer or by immersion of the
                    equipment in cleaning fluids.
    B **False**   A needle shaft within tissues is poorly visualised
                    under ultrasound guidance. However, the needle tip
                    is usually well visualised as a strong echo.
    C **True**
    D **False**   No local anaesthesia is required.
    E **True**   Prophylactic intravenous antibiotics should be given
                    immediately before, and subsequently orally for 3
                    days post-biopsy.

83   In Doppler ultrasound:

A   continuous wave Doppler may be used in fetal heart detection.

B   blood flow within the popliteal vein can be augmented by manual calf compression.

C   the portal vein is best assessed via an anterior approach.

D   the normal velocity waveform of the common carotid artery shows continuous forward flow in diastole.

E   the normal velocity waveform of the external carotid artery may show reversal in diastole.

84   With respect to Doppler imaging of the leg veins:

A   the normal venous flow signal in the legs varies with respiration.

B   compressibility of veins is one of the most reliable signs of patency.

C   an established collateral venous system may simulate flow in a patent major vein.

D   Doppler flow studies are more reliable in detecting thrombus in the veins below the knee than in those above the knee.

E   thrombus may be anechoic.

85   In chest computed tomography (CT):

A   the vagus nerves are commonly visualised.

B   the mediastinal structures are best demonstrated with a narrow window width.

C   the normal pericardium is not visible.

D   normal mediastinal lymph nodes are not visualised.

E   the major fissures are demonstrated as thin white lines in the majority of cases.

83 **A** **True**

  B **True**   This manoeuvre is useful in examination of the deep veins of the leg where normal low velocity blood flow may not otherwise be detected. The Valsalva manoeuvre is also followed by a compensatory transient increase in blood flow in the deep veins of the leg.

  C **False**   An anterior approach to the portal vein is optimal for imaging but provides a poor beam/vessel angle for Doppler studies. In Doppler ultrasound the beam/vessel angle should be no greater than 60°. Therefore, the right lateral intercostal approach optimises the beam/vessel angle.

  D **True**   This is characteristic of a low resistance arterial flow pattern.

  E **True**   This is characteristic of a high resistance arterial flow pattern.

84 **A** **True**   When the patient lies supine, the venous flow signal decreases on inspiration and increases on expiration.

  B **True**   Direct pressure with the ultrasound probe over the vein will cause the normal vein to collapse. If thrombus is present, this will not occur.

  C **True**   Thus causing confusion and inaccuracy.

  D **False**   Duplex Doppler studies have a high degree of accuracy in detecting occlusions in the femoral, popliteal or iliac veins. Below the knee the study is difficult, time consuming and less reliable.

  E **True**   Thus compression studies are important.

85 **A** **False**

  B **True**   A narrow window width (e.g. 300 Hounsfield units) and a soft-tissue level (e.g. 30–50 Hounsfield units) are optimal.

  C **False**   The normal pericardium is visible as a thin stripe of soft tissue density around the heart outlined by mediastinal and epicardial fat.

  D **False**   Normal mediastinal lymph nodes may be visualised. A diameter of 1 cm is considered as the upper limit of a normal node in most parts of the mediastinum.

  E **False**   The major fissures are demonstrated as thin white lines in only 10–20% of CT scans. However their position can be inferred from the relatively avascular plane of lung lying either side of each fissure.

86   When the thorax is examined by high-resolution CT:
   A   contiguous 1 mm thick sections are usually obtained.
   B   the mA is usually increased compared with conventional chest CT.
   C   normal interlobular septa may be visible.
   D   a soft tissue algorithm is used.
   E   motion artefact adjacent to the heart is eliminated.

87   Regarding percutaneous lung biopsy:
   A   a previous contralateral pneumonectomy is a contraindication.
   B   a pneumothorax will be detectable on a chest radiograph in
       approximately 60% of cases.
   C   the risk of pneumothorax is increased if the biopsy needle
       traverses a fissure.
   D   in the case of a large or cavitating lesion it is important to obtain
       material from its margins.
   E   a CT scan is required in all cases to accurately locate the lesion.

88   In CT scanning of the upper abdomen:
   A   the normal spleen enhances irregularly following bolus intravenous
       contrast agents.
   B   the normal gastric wall can be 10 mm thick.
   C   pancreatic examination may require a left lateral decubitus position.
   D   adrenal glands are visualised in approximately 10% of normal
       patients.
   E   the gall bladder wall enhances markedly following intravenous
       contrast enhancement.

89   In CT of the abdomen:
   A   dilute barium can be used to opacify the bowel.
   B   normal intrahepatic bile ducts are usually visible.
   C   oral contrast medium should be given 1 hour prior to the
       examination to produce large bowel opacification.
   D   the diaphragmatic crura can be mistaken for enlarged lymph nodes.
   E   image interpretation is easier in thin rather than obese patients.

86 **A** **False**   1 mm thick sections are usually obtained at intervals from the lung apices to bases.

   B **True**   Increasing mA reduces the visible image noise and improves scan quality.

   C **True**   Normal centrilobular arteries may also be visible. The centrilobular bronchiole is not normally seen.

   D **False**   A bony algorithm is used in high-resolution CT.

   E **False**

87 **A** **True**   Because a pneumothorax would be poorly tolerated.

   B **False**   A chest radiograph demonstrates a pneumothorax in 15–25% of cases. CT shows a much higher percentage (about 60%).

   C **True**   The biopsy needle will be traversing four layers of pleura.

   D **True**   The cells in the centre of the lesion may be necrotic and unrepresentative of its true cytological nature.

   E **False**   The lesion can often be adequately detected using biplane fluoroscopy or a C-arm.

88 **A** **True**   Due to variable rates of blood flow through its pulp.

   B **True**   The normal small bowel wall is up to 3 mm thick. The normal colonic wall is up to 5 mm thick.

   C **False**   In pancreatic CT examination a right lateral decubitus position immediately after oral contrast medium may be helpful in opacifying the duodenum.

   D **False**   Adrenal glands are visualised in almost all normal adults.

   E **True**

89 **A** **True**   Barium concentrations between 1–3% w/v are optimal.

   B **False**   Normal intrahepatic bile ducts are not usually visible on CT.

   C **False**   Oral contrast medium should be given at least 4 hours prior to the examination to produce large bowel opacification. Oral contrast medium should be given gradually over a period of 1 hour before scanning to produce small bowel opacification.

   D **True**

   E **False**   Much of the natural contrast in CT is provided by fat, thus making image interpretation easier in obese patients.

90 In CT of the normal pelvis:

A vaginal tampons should always be removed prior to scanning to avoid confusing artefacts.

B the ovaries are readily identified.

C the paired seminal vesicles have a characteristic bowtie-shaped appearance.

D the spermatic cord is visualised in the inguinal canal.

E the prostate is separated from the bladder by a fat plane.

91 Regarding computed tomography:

A suspended respiration is required for examination of the neck.

B air is seen within the oesophagus in approximately 80% of patients on chest CT.

C filling defects may be seen in the normal superior vena cava during contrast enhancement.

D CT pelvimetry has a much lower radiation dose than conventional pelvimetry.

E patients undergoing a pelvic examination should have a full bladder.

92 In CT examination of the brain:

A most adults' heads are adequately examined in approximately 15 contiguous 10 mm thick axial sections.

B when scanning the posterior cranial fossa bony artefact is reduced by increasing slice thickness.

C intravenous contrast enhancement should precede pituitary fossa examination.

D white matter is more dense than grey matter.

E the internal capsule is of a higher attenuation value than the caudate nuclei.

90 A **False**   A vaginal tampon is indicated in pelvic scanning. Air trapped by the tampon produces negative contrast.
   B **False**   They are difficult to identify on CT.
   C **True**
   D **True**   It is seen as a thin-walled oval structure of fat density containing small dots representing the vas deferens and spermatic vessels.
   E **False**

91 A **False**   Suspended respiration is not required. However, the patient should be asked not to swallow during the exposure.
   B **True**
   C **True**   Filling defects in the superior vena cava result from incomplete mixing of opacified and unopacified blood.
   D **True**   CT pelvimetry measurements are also accurate and reproducible.
   E **True**

92 A **True**   10 mm thick contiguous sections from the posterior arch of the atlas to the vertex.
   B **False**   When scanning the posterior cranial fossa, thinner and more frequent sections will reduce bone artefacts and improve scan quality. Alteration in gantry angulation may also reduce artefact.
   C **True**
   D **False**   White matter is less dense (i.e. has a lower Hounsfield number) than grey matter.
   E **False**   The internal capsule is of a lower attenuation value than the caudate nuclei.

93   In CT scanning of the orbits:

A   the superior ophthalmic vein cannot be distinguished separately from the superior rectus muscle.

B   direct coronal sections are often necessary.

C   intravenous contrast enhancement is mandatory.

D   axial sections are acquired parallel to the neuro-ocular plane.

E   the prone patient position is essential when obtaining direct coronal sections.

94   When imaging the larynx:

A   lateral tomograms give a better demonstration of the vocal cords than anteroposterior (AP) tomograms.

B   phonating "ee" approximates the vocal cords.

C   axial CT sections of 5 mm thickness are technically appropriate.

D   ossification of the laryngeal cartilages is more easily seen on the frontal radiograph than the lateral radiograph.

E   soft tissue discrimination is better on MRI than CT.

95   Dimeglumine gadopentate (Gadolinium):

A   is superparamagnetic.

B   shortens the T1-relaxation time.

C   is excreted by the kidneys.

D   produces a transient increase in serum iron levels following intravenous injection.

E   has no severe adverse effects.

93 A False
   B True   In addition to axial sections. Coronal reformats should be reserved for those patients whose dental fillings make direct coronal sections difficult.
   C False   Intravenous contrast enhancement is generally given to show up space-occupying lesions in better detail or when there is suspicion of intracranial involvement by a lesion. It is not necessary in thyroid eye disease nor following trauma.
   D True
   E False   To obtain direct coronal sections the patient usually lies prone with the chin elevated. However, if this is not possible, then direct coronal sections may be obtained by placing the patient supine with the neck hyperextended.

94 A False   The vocal cords are best seen on AP tomograms.
   B True
   C True
   D False   Laryngeal cartilage ossification is best seen on the lateral radiograph which avoids superimposition of cartilage over spine.
   E True   In addition, the use of coronal and sagittal sections in MRI allows visualisation of the intrinsic laryngeal muscles.

95 A False   Gadolinium is a paramagnetic contrast agent.
   B True   Gadolinium leads to an increased signal on T1-weighted MR images and is therefore known as a positive contrast agent. Superparamagnetic contrast agents reduce the T2-relaxation time, leading to a decreased signal on T2-weighted images. They are known as negative contrast agents.
   C True   It has a plasma half-life of about 90 minutes.
   D True   Therefore serum iron estimations may be inaccurate in the 24 hours following intravenous injection.
   E False   Gadolinium may result in an anaphylactoid reaction. Minor reactions are seen in about 0.14% patients following injection; these include nausea, local burning sensation, urticaria and headache.

96   Regarding spin echo imaging:
  A   structures with a short T1 produce high signal intensity in
      T1-weighted images.
  B   structures with a short T2 produce high signal intensity in
      T2-weighted images.
  C   fat produces a higher signal intensity than muscle on a
      T1-weighted image.
  D   cerebrospinal fluid usually produces a lower signal intensity
      than grey matter on a T2-weighted image.
  E   cortical bone has a high signal intensity on T1- and
      T2-weighted images.

97   Regarding MRI of the brain:
  A   the pituitary gland enhances poorly with intravenous
      Gadolinium.
  B   mascara should be removed prior to the examination.
  C   the paranasal sinus mucosa enhances with intravenous
      Gadolinium.
  D   on T1-weighted images grey matter has a higher signal
      intensity than white matter.
  E   on T2-weighted images white matter has a higher signal than
      grey matter.

**98   A significant deflection (rotational movement as a result of the
      primary field) of the following implants/devices will occur during
      MRI:**
  A   Charnley total hip replacement prosthesis.
  B   Björk-Shiley heart valve replacement.
  C   copper intra-uterine contraceptive device.
  D   dental amalgam.
  E   all surgical clips.

96 A True   Structures with a long T1 produce low signal intensity on T1-weighted images.

    B False Structures with a long T2 produce high signal intensity on T2-weighted images. Structures with short T2 produce low signal intensity on T2-weighted images.

    C True   Fat has a shorter T1 than muscle.

    D False Cerebrospinal fluid usually has a longer T2 than grey matter.

    E False Cortical bone has a low signal intensity on T1- and T2-weighted images.

---

97 A False It enhances strongly.

    B True   Mascara may contain ferromagnetic material and thus cause signal loss/geometric distortion.

    C True

    D False The reverse is true.

    E False The reverse is true.

---

98 A False Most orthopaedic implants do not undergo significant deflection and are therefore safe.

    B False Many modern prosthetic heart valves are submitted to a deflection force which is not clinically significant. However, some prosthetic valves, including the Starr-Edwards valve, may undergo significant deflection.

    C False

    D False

    E False Whether a surgical clip undergoes significant deflection or not depends on the individual type of clip.

99   The following statements regarding MRI are true:

A   the entire scanning suite is designated a controlled area.

B   the noise heard during scanning arises from the transmitted radiofrequency pulses.

C   60% w/v barium is used as a positive bowel contrast agent.

D   Gadolinium enhancement helps to discriminate between recurrent intervertebral disc prolapse and postoperative fibrosis.

E   cardiac gating improves image quality in examination of the cervical spine.

100   In magnetic resonance imaging:

A   T1-weighted spin echo (SE) images usually visualise anatomical structures better than T2-weighted SE images.

B   the signal from fat is suppressed by short T1-Inversion Recovery (STIR) sequences.

C   healthy tendons can acquire abnormally high signal on short TE sequences if orientated at 55° to the static magnetic field.

D   rapidly flowing blood or cerebrospinal fluid usually has high signal on spin echo sequences.

E   regarding magnetic resonance angiography (MRA), the time of flight technique is more sensitive to slow flow than the phase contrast technique.

99 **A** **False**   The area inside the 10 Gauss line is designated as controlled. Any person entering the controlled area should remove all loose ferromagnetic objects susceptible to the missile effect, and any magnetic cards. Persons with pacemakers must not enter.

  B **False**   The noise which is heard during scanning arises from vibration in the gradient coils due to the varying magnetic fields.

  C **False**   Barium is used as a negative bowel contrast agent, by shortening T2 and therefore appearing black on T2-weighted spin echo images. Gadolinium and fatty oils are used as positive bowel contrast agents.

  D **True**   Imaging must be performed shortly after intravenous Gadolinium as fibrous tissue enhances immediately but disc material does not enhance within 10 minutes of injection.

  E **True**   Artefact produced by cerebrospinal fluid pulsation in the cervical spine can be reduced by synchronising data acquisition to the cardiac cycle.

100 **A** **True**   T2-weighted spin echo images usually demonstrate pathology better than T1-weighted SE images.

  B **True**   It is particularly useful in the examination of tissues with a high fat content (e.g. orbit, parotid gland, bone marrow).

  C **True**   This is referred to as the magic angle phenomenon and may mimic pathological tendinous change. The effect is most likely to be seen in curved tendons (e.g. supraspinatus tendon).

  D **False**   In spin echo sequences, rapidly following blood or cerebrospinal fluid usually has low signal. Slow flowing blood usually has high signal. However in gradient echo techniques, virtually all vessels are hyperintense.

  E **False**   The opposite is true. Time of flight (TOF) MRA uses a gradient echo sequence with a flip angle of 30–60° to maximise flow-related enhancement of vessels that occurs due to the entry phenomenon. Thus in-plane flow will produce less signal so that TOF techniques are less sensitive to slow flow within the imaging plane.

3 Physics

1   **Regarding the structure of the atom:**
   A   an electron has a unit negative charge and no mass.
   B   the number of neutrons is the same as the number of orbital electrons in an electrically neutral atom.
   C   the atomic mass (A) of an element is always equal to or greater than its atomic number (Z).
   D   an electron in the K shell has a higher binding energy than an electron in the M shell.
   E   the nuclear forces that are called exchange forces are effective only at very short distances.

2   **Regarding radioactivity:**
   A   the maximum number of electrons in the M shell is 64.
   B   an isobar is any nucleus which contains the same number of protons as another given nucleus.
   C   all isotopes achieve stability by the process of radioactive decay.
   D   the binding energy of an electron in a particular shell increases with an increase in the atomic number.
   E   an alpha particle is four times heavier than an electron.

1 A False An electron has a mass of 9.109×10^{-13} kg.
  B False In an electrically neutral atom, the number of protons is equal to the number of orbital electrons.
  C True The atomic mass of an element is comprised of the number of protons and the number of neutrons present in the nucleus. The atomic mass will therefore always be equal to or greater than the atomic number.
  D True The binding energy is greater for those shells which are closer to the nucleus.
  E True The exchange forces in the nucleus are also called short range forces and are effective at distances of 10^{-15} m.

2 A False Use the $2n^2$ law to calculate the number of electrons allowed in any orbit. Here n is the shell number. The shell number n starts from n = 1 for the K shell.
        K shell, n = 1, number of electrons = 2
        L shell, n = 2, number of electrons = 8
        M shell, n = 3, number of electrons = 18
    The number of electrons in the M shell will be 18 and not 64.
  B False An isobar is any nucleus which has the same atomic mass number as another nucleus.
  C False Not all isotopes are radioactive, e.g. ^{12}C and ^{13}C are isotopes of carbon but neither is radioactive.
  D True The shell radii are smaller with increasing atomic number and the binding energy is greater for those shells closer to the nucleus.
  E False An alpha particle is 7280 times heavier than an electron.

3 Regarding radioactivity:

A the unit of radioactivity is the Becquerel (Bq) where 1 Bq is 1 disintegration per minute.

B the unit of specific activity is Becquerels per millilitre (Bq/ml).

C it is possible to slow the radioactive decay process by lowering the temperature of the radioactive sample to −4°C.

D stable heavy nuclei contain an increased number of neutrons relative to the number of protons.

E gamma rays exceed X-rays in their maximum possible energy.

4 Regarding radioactivity:

A ^{14}C decays to ^{14}N by the process of isomeric transition.

B during positron and electron annihilation two gamma photons of 150 keV energy are emitted.

C during a beta decay the total energy carried by the beta particle and the associated neutrino is constant.

D for ionizing radiations, frequency (ν) multiplied by its wavelength (λ) is always constant.

E the quantum energy (E) associated with the individual X-ray and gamma photons can be calculated by dividing Planck's constant (h) by the frequency of the radiation.

3 A False   1 Bq is equal to 1 disintegration per second.
  B False   Bq/ml is a concentration of radioactivity and not specific activity; the latter is expressed as Bq/kg, i.e. activity per unit mass.
  C False   The radioactive decay process is not affected by the temperature of the sample.
  D True   An increased number of neutrons reduces the extent of repulsive columbic forces between the positively charged protons.
  E True   Gamma rays originate from unstable nuclei and X-rays originate from changes in the electron shells. The maximum amount of energy available during nuclear transformation is much higher than that involved in the electron transfers (Bremsstrahlung).

---

4 A False   Isomeric transitions occur between metastable and stable states, e.g. ^{99m}Tc decays to ^{99}Tc. Note that the metastable state is denoted by the letter m.
  B False   An annihilation process involving a positron and an electron produces two gamma photons of 0.511 MeV energy. This follows the principle of mass and energy equivalence.
  C True   During beta decay the kinetic energy is shared between the beta particle and the neutrino. Therefore the total energy carried by a beta particle and a neutrino for a specific beta transformation is always constant.
  D True   The product of frequency (v) and wavelength (λ) is constant and is equal to the velocity of light c (3×10^8 m^{-1}).
  E False   The electromagnetic radiations can be considered as energy quanta or photons. The energy associated with the photons is given by the following relationship: $E = hv$. The energy is a product of the frequency (v) and Planck's constant (h) 6.63×10^{-34} Js.

5   **Regarding the interaction of electrons with matter:**
   A   electrons travel only a short distance in tissue ranging from a few microns to a few millimetres.
   B   Bremsstrahlung radiation occurs when a low energy electron interacts with matter.
   C   the average energy required to form an ion pair is approximately 10 000 eV.
   D   units of linear energy transfer are expressed as keV μm^{-1}.
   E   a low atomic number material, such as perspex, is more suitable than a high atomic number material, such as lead, for protection against pure beta emitters.

6   **Regarding the attenuation of X- and gamma radiation by matter:**
   A   the linear attenuation coefficient (μ) is the fractional reduction in the monoenergetic photon beam per unit mass.
   B   the half value thickness (HVT) is the thickness of material which will reduce the intensity of the photon beam to 70% of its original value.
   C   under narrow beam conditions, for 100 keV photons, the half value thickness (HVT) for water is less than the half value thickness of lead.
   D   the mass attenuation coefficient is given by the linear attenuation coefficient divided by the density.
   E   six half value layers reduce the photon beam intensity to 1.56% of its original intensity.

7   **Regarding the interaction of X-rays and gamma rays with matter:**
   A   during elastic scattering the photon is deflected from its path and suffers no loss of energy.
   B   the energy of the Compton scattered photon is the same as that of the incident photon.
   C   the attenuation coefficient decreases with increasing energy.
   D   during elastic scattering no ionization occurs.
   E   during Compton scatter the direction of the scattered photon depends on the energy of the incident photon.

8   **Regarding the photoelectric effect:**
   A   an interacting photon disappears completely.
   B   it is an interaction between a photon and a free electron.
   C   it does not produce an ionised atom.
   D   it produces characteristic X-radiations.
   E   no further ionizations or excitations occur in the matter as the photoelectron slows down.

5 A **True**
   B **False** Bremsstrahlung radiation occurs when a high energy electron is de-accelerated by interacting with the electric field of the nucleus.
   C **False** The average energy required to form an ion pair is 34 eV.
   D **True**
   E **True** Bremsstrahlung radiation is dependent on the atomic number of the interacting matter. Therefore a low atomic number material such as perspex should be used as a shielding material for pure high energy beta emitters.

6 A **False** The linear attenuation coefficient is the fractional reduction in the monoenergetic photon beam per unit length.
   B **False** The HVT will reduce the intensity of the photon beam to 50% of its original value.
   C **False** For a given photon energy the value of the HVT is inversely proportional to the atomic number of the material. Water is a low atomic number material and therefore will have a higher value of HVT than lead which is a high atomic number material.
   D **True** This is the definition of mass attenuation coefficient.
   E **True**

7 A **True**
   B **False** The energy of the Compton scattered photon is less than that of the incident photon.
   C **True**
   D **True**
   E **True** Very low energy photons are scattered almost equally in all directions but as the energy increases a greater percentage is scattered in a forward direction.

8 A **True**
   B **False** The interaction is between a photon and a bound electron.
   C **False** A bound electron is ejected during the photoelectric effect resulting in an ionized atom.
   D **True**
   E **False** The photoelectron loses its energy by causing further ionisations and excitations in the matter.

9   **Regarding pair production:**
   A   it is the predominant process of interaction for photons with energies less than 1.02 MeV.
   B   the incoming photon interacts with a free electron to produce an electron-positron pair.
   C   it is an example of creation of mass from energy.
   D   during an annihilation process a positron interacts with an electron to create four 0.51 MeV photons.
   E   the annihilation process is an example of conversion of mass into equivalent energy.

10   **Regarding photon interactions in the patient during diagnostic X-ray imaging:**
   A   they are independent of the kV used.
   B   photon interactions in the soft tissue are mainly scattering events.
   C   the average atomic number of soft tissue is higher than that of bone.
   D   photoelectric absorption is the main attenuation process occuring in bone.
   E   the pair production interaction does not take place.

11   **The following statements are true of the photoelectric effect in diagnostic imaging:**
   A   all the energy of the incident photon is transferred to the orbital electron.
   B   the ejected electron is usually trapped within the electron traps in the soft tissues.
   C   following the ejection of the electron the vacancy created is filled by an outer shell (or valency bond) electron.
   D   it is the means by which aluminium filters remove low energy photons.
   E   it is the predominant mechanism of X-ray interaction with iodinated contrast agents.

9 **A** **False**   Pair production requires the energy of the interacting photon to be more than 1.02 MeV.

    B **False**   Pair production occurs when the photon passes close to a nucleus.

    C **True**

    D **False**   During an annihilation process two 0.51 MeV photons are formed.

    E **True**

---

10 **A** **False**   The nature of the interaction depends on the photon energy and therefore on the kV used.

    B **True**   Compton scatter is the predominant interaction.

    C **False**   The average atomic number of soft tissue is 7.4 and that of bone is 14.0.

    D **True**

    E **True**   Pair production does not take place below 1.02 MeV.

---

11 **A** **True**

    B **False**   The ejected electron loses its kinetic energy as it passes through matter as a result of further interactions with atoms and molecules. After losing all its kinetic energy the electron populates the conduction band.

    C **True**

    D **True**

    E **True**

12 **The following statements are true:**
  A the linear attenuation coefficient is defined as the fractional reduction in the intensity per unit length.
  B the mass attenuation coefficient depends on the density of the interacting medium.
  C the mass attenuation coefficients of 1 g of ice and 1 g of water are the same.
  D the higher attenuation coefficient of muscle compared to that of fat produces enhanced radiographic contrast at low photon energies.
  E minimum X-ray absorption is achieved when the K edge of an absorber is equal to the energy of the X-ray beam.

13 **Regarding the interaction of X-rays with matter:**
  A attenuation in fat is predominantly due to Compton interactions at 60 keV.
  B attenuation in bone is predominantly due to the photoelectric effect at 60 keV.
  C the majority of electrons in the soft tissues may be considered to be free electrons.
  D bone gives rise to more scattered radiation than muscle per unit mass.
  E virtually all of the photon energy is transferred to the ejected electron in a Compton interaction.

14 **The linear attenuation coefficient of an X-ray beam:**
  A is defined as the reduction in intensity per unit length.
  B is higher for bone than for fat at 30 keV.
  C is higher for fat than for bone when Compton interaction predominates.
  D can be used to calculate the half value thickness (HVT) of a material for a given monoenergetic photon beam.
  E is constant for a monoenergetic beam.

12 A True
   B True The mass attenuation coefficient is a ratio of the linear attenuation coefficient and the density of the interacting medium.
   C True The linear attenuation coefficients for water and ice are different (0.214 cm^{-1} and 0.196 cm^{-1} respectively). The densities of water and ice are different (1 g/cm^3 and 0.917 g/cm^3 respectively). Therefore the mass attenuation coefficient for water is $0.214/1 = 0.214$ cm^2/g and that for ice is $0.196/0.917 = 0.214$ cm^2/g.
   D True
   E False This will result in maximum X-ray absorption, since photoelectric absorption is maximal when the X-ray beam energy equals the binding energy of an inner shell electron of the absorber.

---

13 A True In soft tissues Compton interaction is predominant. The photoelectric interaction becomes significant only at very low energies.
   B False The attenuation in bone is predominantly due to Compton scattering at 60 keV. Photoelectric absorption predominates at about 30 keV and below.
   C True
   D False Almost all the scattered radiation at diagnostic energies comes from Compton scatter. Muscles produce more Compton scatter per unit mass than bone in the diagnostic energy range.
   E False The interacting photon retains most of its original energy.

---

14 A False The linear attenuation coefficient is the fractional reduction in intensity per unit length (for an infinitesimally small length).
   B True
   C False It is higher for bone than for fat because of the density effect even when Compton interaction predominates.
   D True The HVT = 0.693/linear attenuation coefficient for a given material and monoenergetic beam combination.
   E True

15   Regarding X-ray production in diagnostic imaging:

A   the filament is raised to incandescence by a high filament current which produces a space charge of protons around the filament by thermionic emission.

B   the filament is made out of tungsten because it is inexpensive and easy to replace.

C   the focusing cup of a cathode is made of a relatively poor thermionic emitter material that has a high melting point.

D   the tube current is measured in milliamperes.

E   over 99% of the energy carried by the electrons is converted into X-rays and less than 1% of the energy is lost as heat.

16   Regarding the X-ray tube used in diagnostic radiography:

A   the focusing cup of the cathode is designed so as to spread the electrons over the entire surface of the anode.

B   the addition of rhenium in a tungsten target makes the target tougher and less likely to crack under the stresses caused by heating.

C   a dual focus tube has two filaments of differing size, which enables the production of two different sizes of electron foci on the anode.

D   the glass envelope is filled with an inert gas such as neon in order to increase heat dissipation during X-ray production.

E   the glass envelope is made of borosilicate.

17   Regarding X-ray production:

A   the filament current is the same as the X-ray tube current.

B   the mA is related to the filament current.

C   a compound anode is usually made of copper and zinc.

D   the electrons from the filament are focused on a target material such as tungsten.

E   the anode angle is the angle between the plane of the cathode filament and the plane of the anode.

15 A **False**   Tho process will produce a space charge of electrons around the filament.
    B **False**   The filament is made of tungsten because it is a good thermionic emitter, does not vaporise easily, and can be readily drawn into a thin coiled wire.
    C **True**   For example nickel.
    D **True**
    E **False**   Less than 1% of the energy carried by the electrons is converted into X-rays and over 99% of the energy is lost as heat.

16 A **False**   The focusing cup is designed so that the electrons are concentrated on a small part of the anode called the focal spot.
    B **True**
    C **True**   The small filament is used for fine focus radiography.
    D **False**   The glass envelope of the X-ray tube is evacuated so as to allow the free movement of electrons from the filament to the anode.
    E **True**

17 A **False**   The filament current and the X-ray tube current are not the same. The filament current is typically of the order of 5 A while a typical X-ray tube current is about 200 mA.
    B **True**   An increase in filament current will result in an increased thermionic emission of electrons and this results in an increase in the tube current.
    C **False**   The anode is usually made of copper and tungsten.
    D **True**
    E **True**   The anode angle varies between 6° and 20°. The smaller the anode angle, the smaller the apparent (or effective) focal spot.

18   Regarding X-ray production:

A   the deceleration of electrons in the target produces X-rays.

B   the processes of Bremsstrahlung radiation and characteristic radiation are involved.

C   the anode heel effect produces a reduction in the X-ray intensity for those X-rays which are emitted from the anode at near-grazing angles to the face of the target.

D   a tube with a fixed anode has better cooling characteristics than one with a rotating anode because more heat is produced during anode rotation.

E   the intensity of an X-ray beam (up to 100 keV) is proportional to the atomic number (Z) of a thin target.

19   Regarding the rating and operation of the X-ray tube:

A   any two X-ray tubes used for similar diagnostic procedures will have identical rating charts.

B   rectification, thermal capacity of the anode, and the anode angle are selectable during the operation of an X-ray tube.

C   the rating of an X-ray tube for fine focus use is lower than that for broad focus use.

D   the rating chart depends on several factors including the kVp used.

E   a rotating anode tube has a significantly higher rating than a tube which uses a stationary anode.

20   Regarding X-ray timers:

A   the timer switch controls the X-ray exposure by controlling the filament current.

B   a thyratron is a gas-filled tube that functions as an electronic switch.

C   mechanical timers are accurate to 0.01 seconds.

D   in electronic timers a resistance-capacitor circuit is used to determine the length of the X-ray exposure.

E   ionisation chambers are not suitable for use as X-ray timers.

18 A **True**
    B **True**
    C **True**
    D **False**   The rotating anode tube has better cooling
                characteristics as the heat generated on the anode is
                spread over a much larger area. Therefore there is a
                greater area available to lose heat.
    E **True**   High atomic number elements such as tungsten
                (Z = 74) are ideal as target materials.

19 A **False**   Each tube has its own rating chart.
    B **False**   These factors are not selectable but are
                predetermined.
    C **True**   The rating of the X-ray tube using the fine focus is
                lower than that when using the broad focus as the
                electron beam is focused onto a smaller area and
                this causes a higher temperature for the same mA.
    D **True**   The rating of an X-ray tube depends on the focal
                spot size, the kVp, the exposure time and the
                rectification.
    E **True**   A rotating anode has more efficient heat loss;
                because of the moving track the energy is deposited
                over a larger area on the anode resulting in a higher
                rating.

20 A **False**   The timer switch controls the X-ray exposure by
                controlling the high voltage supplied to the X-ray
                tube. The filament heats and cools relatively slowly
                and therefore cannot be used to regulate the
                exposure times.
    B **True**   A thyratron is a gas-filled (e.g. low pressure argon)
                triode valve. The potential on the grid is used to
                switch the thyratron on. The thyratron is switched off
                by reducing the anode potential to nearly cathode
                potential so that gas multiplication no longer takes
                place.
    C **False**   Mechanical timers are accurate to only 0.25 seconds.
    D **True**
    E **False**   Ionisation chambers can be used as phototimers.
                They are designed to be as radiolucent as possible
                so that they can be placed in front of the X-ray film.

21 Regarding the focal spot:

   A   a centrally peaked radiation intensity distribution gives a focal spot with improved resolving power.
   B   size increases with an increase in the tube current.
   C   size increases with increasing kVp.
   D   size measurement must be made in the central part of the X-ray beam.
   E   the modulation transfer function (MTF) deteriorates with an increase in the focal spot size.

22 Regarding the focal spot:

   A   true magnification is always smaller than geometric magnification.
   B   star test pattern imaging demonstrates the intensity distribution of radiation from the focal spot.
   C   a pinhole diameter of 0.5 mm is recommended for measurement of a focal spot of less than 1 mm.
   D   star test pattern imaging is generally recommended for assessing focal spot sizes larger than 0.3 mm.
   E   the actual physical size of a focal spot can be directly measured in a star pattern imaging test.

23 Regarding X-ray film:

   A   the silver halides are sensitive in the blue part of the visible spectrum at approximately 480 nm.
   B   the addition of a small amount of silver iodide to silver bromide reduces the sensitivity of the film.
   C   the cut-off sensitivity of an emulsion is the wavelength beyond which the film is no longer sensitive.
   D   the spectral sensitivity of silver halide is altered by adding certain dyes to the emulsions.
   E   an emulsion with a wide range of grain sizes produces a film that has a high film contrast.

21 A True   Geometric uncharpness due to asymmetrical
radiation distribution is thus minimised.
    B True   This effect is called blooming and is more marked at
low kVp and high mAs.
    C False The focal spot size decreases slightly with increasing
kVp.
    D True   The apparent size of the focal spot changes away
from the central ray. The focal spot length is shorter
when measured at the anode end than at the
cathode end of the X-ray beam.
    E True   An increase in the focal spot size increases the
magnification factor which causes deterioration in the
MTF.

22 A False Magnification depends on the focal spot size.
Geometric magnification is calculated assuming that
all X-rays originate from a point source. In reality, the
focal spot has finite dimensions and therefore the
true magnification is always greater than the
geometric magnification.
    B False Star test pattern imaging measures the resolving
capacity of the focal spot. The intensity distribution of
radiation is demonstrated by pinhole imaging.
    C False The recommended diameter is 0.003 mm.
    D False Star pattern imaging is recommended for focal spot
sizes smaller than 0.3 mm as the pinhole image of a
0.3 mm focal spot is difficult to assess without
specialised equipment.
    E False The focal spot size can be derived from the star
pattern imaging test using a formula.

23 A True
    B False The addition of silver iodide increases the film
sensitivity.
    C True
    D True
    E False Such a film is sensitive to a wide range of exposures.
It therefore has a high exposure latitude and a low
film contrast.

24   Regarding X-ray film:

A   the latent image is produced on the film after exposure and development.

B   the latent image is formed by partial reduction of the silver bromide crystals during the exposure.

C   gelatin is used as the basis of the emulsion.

D   there is an excess of silver bromide over silver iodide in the film emulsion.

E   the speed of an emulsion is largely dependent on the range of grain sizes (grain size distribution).

25   Regarding sensitometry:

A   the transmission ratio is the ratio of transmitted to incident light (i.e. I_t/I_o).

B   the opacity is the reciprocal of the transmission ratio (i.e. I_o/I_t).

C   the optical density is an antilog value of the opacity.

D   the density is linearly related to the weight of the film silver.

E   the characteristic curve of a film is a plot of optical density (D) against relative exposure (E).

26   Regarding X-ray film:

A   the normal density due to the base plus fog of a correctly stored unexposed film is approximately 1.

B   ageing of the film decreases the overall level of base plus fog.

C   the base plus fog level is independent of the processor temperature.

D   density is proportional to the logarithm of film exposure in the linear part of the characteristic curve of the film.

E   the greater the exposure range over which the density (D) versus relative log exposure (log E) is linear, then the greater is the latitude of the film.

24 A False   The latent image is formed after exposure and before development.

    B True

    C True   These are some of the reasons why gelatin is used: when the silver halide is formed the gelatin keeps the grains dispersed; gelatin forms a flexible transparent layer; gelatin protects the latent image.

    D True   Film emulsion contains grains of silver halide — approximately 90% silver bromide and 10% silver iodide.

    E False   The speed of an emulsion is largely dependent on the average size of the grains. The larger the average grain size, the greater the speed of the emulsion.

---

25 A True   A perfectly opaque area has a zero transmission ratio. A perfectly transparent area has a transmission ratio of one.

    B True   A perfectly transparent area of an image has an opacity of one. A perfectly opaque area has an infinite opacity. The blackest part of a radiographic image has an opacity approaching 10 000.

    C False   The optical density is a log value of the opacity.

    D True

    E False   The characteristic curve is a plot of optical density (D) against the log of the relative exposure (log E).

---

26 A False   The density due to base plus fog for these conditions is approximately 0.2.

    B False   The level of base plus fog increases with ageing.

    C False   The level of base plus fog increases with an increase in the processor temperature.

    D True   The average slope of the linear part of the characteristic curve gives the gamma of the film.

    E True   The greater the film latitude, the lower the film gamma and vice versa.

27 Radiographic contrast depends on the:
  A   inherent contrast of the film.
  B   development conditions of the film.
  C   contrast of the subject.
  D   viewing conditions of the film.
  E   basic fog.

28 Regarding processing of X-ray films:
  A   the developer has a pH range between 11 and 13.
  B   the fixer has a pH of 7.
  C   the developer precipitates the metallic silver from the bromide, chloride and iodide salts.
  D   the numerical value of the amplification gain achieved by the process of developing is 10^2.
  E   the fixer contains ammonium thiosulphate.

29 Regarding film processor monitoring:
  A   the base plus fog level is estimated by measuring the density of the most exposed part of the film.
  B   the film processor performance should be assessed once a week.
  C   the film speed and the film contrast should be measured daily.
  D   the film processor should be monitored at a regular time during the day.
  E   the films which are used for monitoring film processors should be taken from a specially reserved film box.

27 A **True**   The inherent contrast of the film is determined
                during the manufacture of the emulsion by the size
                and size distribution of the grains of silver halide.
    B **True**
    C **True**   Subject contrast can be influenced by several factors
                of which kV, scattered radiation and intensifying
                screens are the most important.
    D **True**
    E **True**   The overall effect of a high basic fog (base plus fog)
                on a normally exposed radiograph is to reduce the
                radiographic contrast.

28 A **False**   Developers have a pH range between 9.6 and 10.6.
    B **False**   The fixer has a pH range between 4.2 and 4.9.
    C **True**
    D **False**   The amplification gain achieved is much higher, i.e.
                10^9.
    E **True**

29 A **False**   The measurement is made on an unexposed part of
                the film.
    B **False**   The film processor performance should be checked
                daily.
    C **True**
    D **True**   This is essential in order to achieve reproducibility of
                the results.
    E **True**

30   Regarding silver conservation:

   A the electrolytic method produces 50–70% pure silver.

   B in high current density electrolytic units the fixer solution is kept under constant agitation.

   C the silver content of a fixer solution can be estimated by a simple test paper.

   D around 10–20% of the available silver is recoverable by using a metal exchange method.

   E fitting metal exchange units in tandem improves the overall silver recovery efficiency.

31   The following statements are true regarding film/screen combinations:

   A after X-ray exposure, the film produces an image which results from light and direct X-rays in equal proportions.

   B 95% of the X-ray beam is absorbed by the photoelectric effect within the intensifying screen.

   C during the process of fluorescence the phosphor absorbs long wavelength radiations and emits short wavelength radiations.

   D modern film–screen combinations have a resolution range between 200 and 300 line pairs mm^{-1}.

   E the speed of rare earth phosphors is independent of the kVp.

32   Regarding intensifying screens:

   A intensifying screens reduce the amount of scattered radiation.

   B calcium tungstate produces light with a peak wavelength of about 700 nanometres during fluorescence.

   C the intrinsic efficiency of the phosphor is defined as the number of light photons produced per unit area (photons cm^{-2}).

   D approximately half the generated light reaches the film and the rest is absorbed in the screen.

   E the intensification factor of the screen is the ratio of the X-ray exposures needed to produce the same density on a film with and without the screen.

30 A **False**   The electrolytic method produces 95–98% pure silver.
    B **True**   The agitation of the solution brings fresh silver ions
                    close to the surface of the cathode and speeds up the
                    rate of deposition of metallic silver. This allows the
                    use of a higher current and a smaller surface area
                    cathode without the danger of sulphiding, which can
                    eventually stop the plating process altogether.
                    Sulphiding describes the decomposition of the fixer
                    by unused current in the cathode. The products of
                    this decomposition react with any silver ions present
                    in the fixer to form a silver sulphide precipitate,
                    which turns the cathode deposit black.
    C **True**
    D **False**   The metal exchange method is 70% efficient in
                    practice.
    E **True**

31 A **False**   The majority (95%) of the image is produced by light.
                    The rest of the image is formed by the direct action
                    of the X-rays on the film.
    B **True**
    C **False**   During the process of fluorescence the phosphor
                    absorbs short wavelength radiations (X-rays) and
                    emits long wavelength radiations (light).
    D **False**   The resolution range is 2–15 line pairs mm^{-1}.
    E **False**   The speed of rare earth phosphors depends on the
                    kVp. The rare earth screens show maximum speed at
                    80 kVp. Lower speeds occur at both low and high
                    kilovoltages.

32 A **False**   Intensifying screens are used to convert relatively
                    few absorbed X-ray photons into many light photons.
                    Thus the X-ray dose to the patient is reduced while
                    still allowing a properly exposed X-ray film.
    B **False**   The peak wavelength of the light produced is about
                    430 nm and lies in the blue region of the visible
                    spectrum (wavelength range 350–580 nm).
    C **False**   The intrinsic efficiency is defined as the ratio of the
                    light energy liberated by the crystal to the X-ray
                    energy absorbed. The intrinsic efficiency of calcium
                    tungstate is approximately 5%.
    D **True**
    E **True**

33 Regarding intensifying screens:

   A the rare earth phosphors fluoresce maximally in the pure state.
   B the X-ray to light conversion efficiency of rare earth phosphors is the same as that of calcium tungstate ($CaWO_4$).
   C the K edges of barium, lanthanum and gadolinium correspond closely to the maximum intensity of diagnostic X-rays in the primary beam.
   D as a result of fluorescence the terbium-activated gadolinium oxysulphide phosphor produces a continuous spectrum of light with a maximum peak at 430 nm.
   E the rare earth screens show maximum speed at about 80 kVp.

34 Regarding intensifying screens:

   A the speed of the calcium tungstate screen and its ability to record detail have a reciprocal relationship.
   B the ability of phosphors to fluoresce is independent of the ambient temperature.
   C they should be cleaned at regular intervals with an antistatic compound and a detergent applied gently with a lint-free cloth.
   D the film cassette should be checked for good screen-film contact at regular intervals.
   E the intensification factor of calcium tungstate increases with an increase in the kVp of the X-ray beam.

35 Regarding grids used in diagnostic radiography:

   A they are used to improve contrast.
   B they consist of lead foil strips separated by calcium tungstate spacers.
   C the grid ratio is defined as the ratio between the total area covered by the lead foil strips and the total area covered by the interspacing material.
   D the grid ratio of a crossed grid is equal to the average of the ratios of the two superimposed linear grids.
   E a linear grid allows the operator to angle the X-ray tube along the length of the grid without loss of primary radiation.

33 A **False**   The rare earth phosphors, such as gadolinium
                     oxysulphide, fluoresce maximally when atoms of
                     terbium (0.3%) are incorporated to activate the
                     gadolinium oxysulphide.

    B **False**   The X-ray to light conversion efficiency of $CaWO_4$ is
                     approximately 5% while that of the rare earth
                     phosphors is approximately 20%.

    C **True**   Barium K edge 37.4 keV; lanthanum K edge 38.9 keV;
                     gadolinium K edge 50.2 keV.

    D **False**   The spectral emission of this phosphor is due to the
                     terbium ion. Therefore it is not a continuous
                     spectrum but is concentrated in narrow lines with a
                     strong peak at 544 nm.

    E **True**

34 A **True**
    B **False**   Intensifying screens fluoresce more brilliantly at
                     lower temperatures. A higher ambient temperature
                     would require an increase in the exposure factors in
                     order to produce a film with the same optical density.

    C **True**   It is important to keep the intensifying screens clean.
                     Any foreign material on the screen will block light
                     photons and produce an area of underexposure on
                     the film. Regular cleaning with an antistatic and
                     detergent compound should eliminate this problem.

    D **True**   The cassette in which the intensifying screen is
                     mounted holds the film in tight contact with the
                     screen over its entire surface. With a poor screen–film
                     contact the light produced in the intensifying screen
                     will diffuse before it reaches the film and result in
                     unsharpness of the radiographic image.

    E **True**   High kVp X-rays are more abundantly absorbed by
                     the photoelectric process in calcium tungstate
                     screens. This results in a high intensification factor.

35 A **True**   Grids improve contrast by absorbing scattered
                     radiation before it reaches the film.

    B **False**   A grid consists of a series of lead foil strips separated
                     by X-ray transparent spacers. The interspaces are
                     filled with aluminium or an organic compound.

    C **False**   The grid ratio is defined as the ratio between the
                     height of the lead strips and the distance between
                     them.

    D **False**   The grid ratio of a crossed grid is equal to the sum of
                     the ratios of the two linear grids.

    E **True**

36 Regarding a grid:

A   the grid ratio is defined as a ratio of the height of the lead
    strips to their width.
B   the lead strips are approximately 1 mm thick.
C   a measure of primary beam transmission is used in the
    evaluation of grid performance.
D   Bucky factor is used as a measure of the ability of the grid to
    remove scatter.
E   use of a grid is the most important method of improving
    radiographic contrast.

37 Regarding grids used in diagnostic radiography:

A   those with a low grid ratio are more efficient in removing
    scattered radiation than those with a high grid ratio.
B   the primary transmission (Tp) of a grid is inversely
    proportional to its grid ratio.
C   the measured primary transmission is always less than the
    calculated primary transmission.
D   the primary transmission (Tp) is the same as the Bucky factor
    of the grid.
E   the Bucky factor increases with an increase in the grid ratio.

36 **A** **False**   Grid ratio is defined as the ratio between the height of the strips and the distance between them.

  B **False**   The lead strips are approximately 0.05 mm thick.

  C **True**

  D **True**   The Bucky factor is the ratio of the incident radiation falling on the grid to the transmitted radiation passing through the grid. It is a measure of the ability of the grid to remove scatter.

  E **False**   Contrast improvement depends on various factors such as kVp, field size and patient thickness. The use of a grid is one of the means of improving radiographic contrast by reducing the scattered radiation.

37 **A** **False**   Grids with a higher grid ratio have relatively taller lead strips and shorter distances between the lead strips making them more efficient in removing scattered radiation.

  B **True**

  C **True**   The difference is mainly due to some absorption of the primary radiation by the interspace material.

  D **False**   The primary transmission (Tp) indicates the amount of primary radiation absorbed by the grid while the Bucky factor indicates the amount of absorption of both primary and secondary radiation.

  E **True**   High-ratio grids absorb more scattered radiation and have larger Bucky factors than low-ratio grids.

38 Regarding grids:

A the contrast improvement factor (K) is usually determined at 70 kVp by utilising a small field and scatter free conditions.

B the higher the Bucky factor, the greater the exposure factors and radiation dose to the patient.

C the contrast improvement factor (K) remains constant for all grids.

D grid cutoff is the loss of primary radiation that occurs when the images of lead strips are projected wider than they would be with ordinary magnification.

E grid cutoff caused by lateral decentring of the grid is best identified by close inspection of the film under a bright light.

39 Regarding filtration in diagnostic radiography:

A it is the process of increasing the mean energy of polychromatic radiation by passing it through an absorber.

B the process of beam filtration does not reduce the patient dose.

C the inherent filtration of a typical diagnostic tube varies between 0.5 and 1.0 mm of lead.

D the beryllium window X-ray tube designed for soft tissue radiography has a minimum inherent filtration.

E the glass envelope alone is responsible for the inherent filtration of a typical diagnostic X-ray tube.

38 **A** **False** The contrast improvement factor is dependent on kVp, field size and patient or phantom thickness — these three factors determine the amount of scattered radiation. To permit comparison between different grids, the contrast improvement factor is usually determined at 100 kVp with a large field and a 20 cm thick phantom.

   B **True** If the Bucky factor for a particular grid-energy combination is 3, then exposure factors and patient exposure both increase by a factor of 3 above that which would be necessary for the same examination without that grid.

   C **False** The contrast improvement factor increases with an increase in the lead content of the grid.

   D **True**
   E **False** During grid cutoff caused by lateral decentring all the lead strips cut off the same amount of primary radiation. This results in a uniform loss of transmitted radiation over the entire surface of the grid and thus produces a uniformly underexposed radiograph.

---

39 **A** **True**
   B **False** The process of beam filtration removes the low energy photons from the X-ray beam. The low energy photons do not contribute to the radiographic image and their removal by the process of filtration therefore reduces the total patient radiation dose.

   C **False** The inherent filtration of a diagnostic X-ray tube is measured in aluminium equivalent, which is the thickness of aluminium that would produce the same degree of attenuation as the thickness of the material. It usually varies between 0.5 and 1.0 mm of aluminium.

   D **True**
   E **False** The insulating oil surrounding the X-ray tube and the window in the tube housing, as well as the glass envelope, are responsible for the inherent filtration of a typical diagnostic X-ray tube.

40   Regarding filters used in diagnostic radiography:

    A copper and aluminium are the materials of choice for added filtration of the X-ray beam.

    B copper is always used in combination with aluminium as a filter material.

    C in a compound filter the higher atomic number material filter faces the patient and the lower atomic number material filter faces the X-ray tube.

    D the characteristic radiation produced by an aluminium filter can give a significant radiation dose to the skin.

    E an added filter of aluminium 3 mm thick is advantageous over an aluminium filter 2 mm thick.

41   Regarding the air gap technique used in diagnostic radiography:

    A scattered radiation is decreased mainly as a result of filtration caused by the air gap.

    B there is a strong bias for forward scattering in the diagnostic energy range.

    C more scattered radiation reaches the film from the scattering events which occur near the entry surface rather than the exit surface of the patient.

    D a larger air gap is desirable when imaging a thicker part of the body.

    E image sharpness deteriorates with an increase in the air gap unless the focal-film distance is also increased.

40 A True   See answer (C).
  B True   See answer (C).
  C False   Most filtration occurs in the higher atomic number material (copper) and the purpose of the lower atomic number material (aluminium) is to absorb the characteristic radiation from the former. Therefore in a compound filter copper (atomic number 29) always faces the X-ray tube and aluminium (atomic number 13) faces the patient.
  D False   The characteristic radiation produced by aluminium has a very low energy (1.5 keV) which is absorbed in the air gap between the patient and the filter.
  E False   An aluminium filter 2mm thick absorbs most of the photons with energies less than 20 keV. Increasing the filter thickness to 3 mm of aluminium does not offer any further advantage. The excess filtration will cause overall attenuation of the beam without significantly altering the quality of the beam.

---

41 A False   Scattered radiation is reduced because scattered photons miss the film. Very small quantities of radiation are absorbed in the air gap without appreciable beam hardening.
  B False   No forward scattering bias exists. At the energies involved, a photon is likely to scatter in almost any direction equally.
  C False   Most of the scattered photons reaching the film arise near the exit surface of the patient due to a greater angle of capture and less tissue attenuation.
  D True   The ratio of scattered to primary radiation for a given thickness of an absorber depends on the size of the air gap present. A large air gap will reduce the ratio of scattered to primary radiation.
  E True   An increase in the focal-film distance compensates for the greater magnification produced by an increase in the air gap.

42   The following statements are true regarding noise in images produced by a film–screen combination:

A   the image quality of low contrast images is seriously affected by noise.

B   images of comparable optical density contain less noise if rare earth screens are used rather than calcium tungstate screens.

C   the noise decreases as the mean number of X-ray photons that are utilised in the formation of the image increases.

D   an increase in the phosphor thickness will increase the noise to produce a given optical density.

E   the main factor determining the noise is the number of X-ray photons utilised by the screen.

43   Regarding radiographic mottle:

A   structure mottle is caused by defects in the intensifying screens.

B   film graininess makes a significant contribution to the radiographic mottle observed in clinical radiology.

C   quantum mottle is caused by statistical fluctuations in the number of X-ray quanta absorbed per unit area of the intensifying screen.

D   quantum mottle increases with an increase in the number of X-ray quanta used.

E   quantum mottle will be greater with a high kVp.

44   Regarding the radiographic image:

A   parallax unsharpness is seen with the use of single emulsion film.

B   the edge gradient is the region of partial illumination that surrounds the complete shadow.

C   the width of the penumbra is less on the anode side than on the cathode side.

D   absorption unsharpness is greatest in objects with sharp edges.

E   motion unsharpness is increased with shorter exposure times.

42 A True   In low contrast images the density difference
between adjacent structures is less. An increase in
the noise can mask the difference in contrast and
thus reduce image quality.

B False   Lower exposures are used with rare earth screens
and thus noise is increased.

C True
D False   With an increase in the phosphor thickness the noise
will be unchanged as the number of photons used by
the screen remain the same due to the reduced
exposure.

E True

---

43 A True
B False   Film graininess is visible only when radiographic film
is examined with a lens to produce a magnification
of × 5 to × 10. Under normal viewing conditions film
graininess does not make a significant contribution to
the mottle.

C True
D False   Quantum mottle increases with a reduction in the
number of X-ray quanta used. Quantum mottle
decreases with an increase in the number of X-ray
quanta used.

E True   A high kVp will produce a higher intensification
factor and therefore quantum mottle will be greater.

---

44 A False   Parallax unsharpness is produced by the formation of
two images on a double emulsion film where the
emulsions are separated by the width of the film
base.

B True
C True   The orientation of the anode angle produces less
penumbra on the anode side.

D False   The absorption unsharpness is greatest for round or
oval objects. This type of unsharpness arises from
the gradual change in the X-ray absorption across
the boundary.

E False   Motion unsharpness is minimised by reducing
exposure times. Patient immobilisation and organ
compression devices also help to reduce motion
unsharpness.

45 Regarding resolution:

A   the resolution of a film–screen combination is expressed by the number of line pairs per millimetre.

B   the line spread function (LSF) of an X-ray film exposed without a screen is very wide.

C   a system with high resolving power is able to record separate images of small objects placed very close together.

D   in a resolution test object a line pair refers to a pair of adjacent lead strips.

E   in a 4 line pair per mm test object the width of an individual lead strip is 0.25 mm.

46 The modulation transfer function (MTF):

A   is expressed as the number of line pairs per mm.

B   provides an objective measurement of resolution.

C   can be understood as a ratio of the information recorded and the information available.

D   is normally greater than 1.

E   can be calculated from the corresponding line spread function (LSF) data.

47 Regarding modulation transfer function (MTF):

A   the MTF of a film–screen combination may be assessed by imaging a grating.

B   MTF curves can be used to compare image qualities of competing systems.

C   resolving power can be considered to be a single specified point on the MTF curve for use in the comparison of different imaging systems.

D   a 30% response on the MTF curve corresponds approximately to the resolving power of an imaging system.

E   the total MTF of a cascaded system is obtained by adding the individual MTF components.

45 A True
   B False   The LSF is the profile of the intensity curve obtained by collimating the X-ray beam through a very narrow slit. The LSF of an X-ray film exposed without a screen is very narrow as there is no diffusion of X-rays in the film.

   C True
   D False   A line pair refers to a single lead strip and a space of non-absorbing material.

   E False   The width of the lead strip will be 0.125 mm.

---

46 A False   MTF is a function expressing the ratio of amplitudes of spatial frequency under different conditions. It has no units.

   B True
   C True
   D False   The recorded information is normally never greater than the available information and therefore MTF is normally less than 1.

   E True   The mathematical operation known as Fourier transformation is used to derive the MTF from the corresponding LSF data.

---

47 A True   Different methods of evaluating the MTF exist. These are based on exposures of slits or gratings followed by analysis using a microdensitometer.

   B True
   C True
   D False   The resolving power of a system corresponds approximately to the 10% response on the MTF curve.

   E False   The total MTF is a product of the individual MTF components.

48   In an image intensifier:

A   the fluoroscopic X-ray tube is operated at a much lower tube current compared with that used in conventional radiography.

B   the input fluorescent phosphor is made of calcium tungstate.

C   the distance between the input screen and the photocathode is about 1 cm.

D   the photocathode absorbs electrons and emits visible light.

E   the anode has a positive potential of approximately 1500 kV.

49   Regarding image intensifiers:

A   the output fluorescent phosphor is made of caesium iodide.

B   a layer of aluminium is coated on the inner surface of the output phosphor to increase its mechanical strength.

C   the aluminium layer removes spent electrons from the output phosphor screen.

D   the conversion factor is the ratio of the luminescence of the input phosphor to the input exposure rate.

E   in general the overall brightness gain of modern image intensifiers is between 50 and 100.

50   Regarding image intensifiers:

A   output is usually viewed directly by a television camera.

B   the superior image quality of caesium iodide phosphors is due to its greater packing density and higher effective atomic number.

C   unequal magnification across the output fluorescent screen causes an increase in brightness at the periphery.

D   the contrast ratio of an image intensifier is typically measured using an aluminium disc.

E   the image distortion of an image intensifier is assessed using a rectangular grid.

48 A True
   B False   The input screen phosphor is made of caesium iodide.
   C False   The distance between the input screen and the photocathode is only a fraction of a millimetre. This proximity is essential to minimise loss of resolution.
   D False   The photocathode absorbs light photons and emits photoelectrons.
   E False   The anode has a positive potential of approximately 25 kV.

49 A False   The output fluorescent screen phosphor is made of silver activated zinc cadmium sulphide.
   B False   The thin aluminium layer prevents light from travelling back through the tube and reactivating the photocathode.
   C True   Thus avoiding a build up of negative charge.
   D False   It is the ratio of luminescence of the output phosphor to the input exposure rate.
   E False   The overall brightness gain is more than 1000.

50 A True   A television viewing system has several advantages which include production of adequate light output from the television monitor to allow cone vision of an amplified image. It is also a very efficient system because it results in minimal loss of information, and the video signal can be recorded giving a permanent record of the investigation.
   B True
   C False   The brightness at the periphery is reduced and so causes vignetting.
   D False   The contrast ratio of an image intensifier is typically measured using a lead disc which has a diameter 10% that of the image intensifier. The contrast ratio is determined by measuring the light output of the output phosphor with and without the lead disc placed at the centre of the image intensifier.
   E True

51 In a TV camera:

   A the fluoroscopic image from the intensifier is focused on to the Vidicon target using an electronic focusing system.

   B focusing and deflecting coils control the electron beam of the Vidicon tube.

   C the antimony trisulphide globules are in direct contact with the signal plate.

   D the end plate of the anode is a wire mesh which allows the electron beam to reach the target.

   E the antimony trisulphide matrix converts the fluoroscopic optical image into an electrostatic image.

52 Regarding digital subtraction angiography (DSA):

   A the analogue–digital converter (ADC) converts the digital voltage output of the video camera into a range of analogue signals.

   B the analogue–digital conversion for the entire video image is carried out in real time.

   C the subtraction process improves anatomical detail.

   D the video cameras which are used characteristically exhibit a significant amount of lag.

   E Plumbicon cameras utilise lead oxide (PbO) as the target material.

53 Regarding subtraction techniques used in diagnostic radiography:

   A an image without contrast medium is electronically added to an image with contrast medium.

   B an image with contrast medium is known as the subtraction mask.

   C there must be almost perfect registration in order to obtain good subtraction.

   D pixel shifting is a form of post-processing that can be used to eliminate motion artefact.

   E when used in angiography the vessels filled with contrast medium appear black on the subtracted image.

51 A **False** The fluoroscopic image is focused on to the Vidicon target using an optical system.

B **True**

C **False** The antimony trisulphide globules are insulated from the signal plate by a mica matrix.

D **True**

E **True**

52 A **False** The ADC converts analogue signals from the video camera into a range of digital numbers.

B **True**

C **False** DSA improves vascular detail by employing the process of digital subtraction of other anatomical details.

D **False** Lag is not desirable in video cameras used in DSA. It is important to reduce the lag so as to reduce the motion artefacts which are caused by the rapidly changing image as the contrast bolus passes through the vessels.

E **True** PbO exhibits low lag properties.

53 A **False** An image without contrast medium is electronically subtracted from a subsequent post-contrast image.

B **False** A subtraction mask is a pre-contrast image.

C **True** There should be perfect superimposition of structures between the pre- and post-contrast images. Any movement between the two images produces registration artefacts and degrades the resultant image.

D **True** This involves moving one image either horizontally or vertically in order to improve the alignment of two images prior to digital subtraction.

E **True**

54 Regarding dental radiography:

A   it is a high frequency and high dose technique.

B   the voltage across the X-ray tube should be less than 50 kV.

C   a typical dose from a single pantomographic exposure is approximately 1 mSv.

D   equipment used for intra-oral films must be fitted with a field defining spacer cone.

E   for equipment working up to 60 kV the cone must ensure a minimum focus to skin distance of 10 cm.

55 In mammography:

A   a high energy X-ray spectrum is employed in order to visualise structures of low contrast.

B   the mammography unit is usually operated at 80 kVp voltage.

C   the X-ray beam used in mammography using molybdenum as a target consists almost entirely of Bremsstrahlung radiation.

D   the K-characteristic radiation of a molybdenum target forms an intense band between 17.9 keV and 19.5 keV.

E   a double-sided emulsion film-screen combination is used to reduce radiation dose to the breast.

56 Regarding mammography:

A   for magnification mammography a focal spot size of less than 0.2 mm diameter is required.

B   the total permanent filtration of the X-ray tube should not be less than 2.5 mm of aluminium.

C   the window of the X-ray tube is made of thin borosilicate glass.

D   the X-ray tube voltage should be accurate to ±10 kV.

E   the mean glandular dose increases with the use of a scatter grid.

54 A False   Dental radiography is a high frequency but low dose technique.
   B False   The voltage across the X-ray tube is typically 70 kV.
   C False   The dose is approximately 0.08 mSv.
   D True   In order to reduce radiation dose.
   E True   In order to reduce the skin dose.

55 A False   The connective tissue, glandular tissue, skin and fat have very similar attenuation coefficients and thus produce little subject contrast. To visualise structures of low contrast a low energy spectrum is used.
   B False   The maximum tube voltage for mammography is about 30 kVp.
   C False   With lower atomic number target materials the Bremsstrahlung production is less efficient. The mammography X-ray tubes are operated at low voltages. The combination of low atomic number anode and low tube voltage reduces the efficiency of Bremsstrahlung production and characteristic radiation becomes dominant.
   D True
   E False   A single-sided emulsion film and single screen combination is used to maximise resolution. A single-sided emulsion film eliminates parallax; and the single screen is positioned behind the film as this causes slightly less loss in resolution than if placed in front of the film.

56 A True   A focal spot size in the range of 0.2–0.5 mm is used for standard mammography.
   B False   The total filtration of a mammography X-ray tube should not be less than 0.5 mm of aluminium or 0.03 mm of molybdenum.
   C False   The window of the X-ray tube should be made of beryllium with a maximum thickness of 1 mm. Beryllium is the material of choice due to its low atomic number.
   D False   The tube voltage for mammography should be accurate to ±1 kV.
   E True   Higher exposures will be needed with the use of a scatter grid.

57 Regarding linear tomography:

   A the X-ray tube and film are connected by a rigid rod which rotates about a fulcrum.

   B the amplitude of tube travel is measured in centimetres.

   C the plane of interest is positioned approximately 10 cm below the fulcrum.

   D the extent of blurring of an image point is proportional to the distance between that point and the fulcrum plane.

   E the X-ray tube and film move in the same direction.

---

58 Regarding linear tomography:

   A the exposure angle and the tomographic angles are always equal.

   B the blur width is directly proportional to the amplitude of the tube travel.

   C the orientation of the object does not affect the extent of blurring.

   D the blur margin produced by a linear motion tomogram is less sharp than the one produced by a circular motion tomogram.

   E section thickness is directly proportional to the amplitude of X-ray tube travel.

---

59 In computed tomography the following statements are true:

   A the X-ray tube is typically operated at about 70 kVp.

   B filtered back projection is the most common image reconstruction technique utilised in the most modern scanners.

   C the average energy of the emerging beam is significantly lower than that of the incident beam.

   D gas detectors are filled with an inert gas such as xenon at atmospheric pressure.

   E the detectors are mass-produced in order to ensure identical sensitivities.

57 **A** **True**

 B **False**   The amplitude of tube travel is measured in degrees and is called the tomographic arc.

 C **False**   The plane of interest is positioned at the same level as the fulcrum. The plane of interest remains in focus while planes above and below are blurred.

 D **True**

 E **False**   When the X-ray tube moves in one direction the film moves in the opposite direction.

---

58 **A** **False**   Occasionally X-rays are not emitted during part of the tube travel, in which case the tomographic angle is greater than the exposure angle.

 B **True**   The blur width refers to the distance over which the image of an object is spread out on the film.

 C **False**   When the longitudinal axis of a long and narrow organ is orientated in the same direction as the X-ray tube travel, the image is not blurred even if it is lying outside the focal plane.

 D **True**   With linear motion tomography the entire image is uniformly blurred and fades off gradually at its edge. With circular motion tomography the blurred image is not uniform and the margin appears sharper.

 E **False**   An inverse relationship exists between the section thickness and the amplitude of tube travel. i.e. the larger the tomographic angle the thinner the section.

---

59 **A** **False**   The X-ray tube is typically operated at about 120 kVp.

 B **False**   Analytical methods have superseded iterative or back projection methods of image reconstruction.

 C **False**   A photon loses only a small amount of its energy during Compton interaction which is predominant in the CT energy range.

 D **False**   The gas detectors are filled with an inert gas at a high pressure of about 25 atmospheres to increase the detector efficiency.

 E **False**   The detectors do not need to be perfectly matched as the sensitivities are calibrated during imaging.

60 Regarding detectors used in computed tomography:

  A sodium iodide detectors are 60% efficient in the diagnostic X-ray range.

  B bismuth germinate detectors are used in preference to sodium iodide detectors because they are cheaper.

  C the voltage between the electrodes is set high enough to produce an avalanche effect in gas detectors during radiation detection.

  D gas-filled detectors are more efficient than sodium iodide detectors.

  E gas detectors have a linear response which is not affected by the intensities used.

61 Regarding computed tomography:

  A a first generation CT scanner is less efficient in eliminating scattered radiation than a third generation CT scanner.

  B energy discriminators are used to eliminate scattered radiation.

  C detector collimation is the only method of controlling scattered radiation.

  D detector collimators regulate the thickness of the tomographic section.

  E the long axis (cathode–anode) of the X-ray tube is perpendicular to the fan beam.

62 In computed tomography:

  A each square element in the image matrix is called a pixel.

  B a voxel represents a group of four adjacent pixels.

  C the size of a pixel is controlled by detector collimation.

  D the size of a voxel is determined by the width of the X-ray beam.

  E a weighting factor is applied during image reconstruction so as to compensate for the difference between the size and shape of the scanning beam and the picture matrix.

60 A False   Sodium iodide detectors are almost 100% efficient in the diagnostic X-ray range.
    B False   Bismuth germinate detectors are superior to sodium iodide detectors as they have higher efficiency and no afterglow.
    C False   The voltage in ionisation chambers is adjusted such that it does not cause an avalanche but is such that the resultant current is proportional to the energy of absorbed X-rays.
    D False   Gas-filled detectors are less efficient due to their low density compared with that of sodium iodide detectors.
    E True

---

61 A False   A first generation scanner uses a pencil beam source-detector geometry which is more efficient in eliminating scatter than is the fan beam geometry which is employed in third generation scanners.
    B False   The CT X-ray beam is polychromatic and the photons lose a very small amount of energy due to Compton scatter; therefore, a discriminating window would not be useful in eliminating scattered radiation.
    C True
    D True
    E True   This arrangement eliminates the asymmetry in the X-ray output caused by the heel effect.

---

62 A True   A typical image matrix is made up of 256×256 pixels.
    B False   A voxel represents a unit volume of tissue sampled.
    C False   The size of an image pixel is determined by the computer programme.
    D True
    E True

63 Regarding the CT number:

A   it represents a relationship between the linear attenuation coefficient in a pixel and that of its immediate neighbours.

B   it represents the linear attenuation coefficient in each pixel.

C   it is derived by using a magnification factor (K) of 1000 or more.

D   to image materials which have a higher linear attenuation coefficient than bone it is necessary to utilise a higher CT number.

E   it can represent variations of linear attenuation coefficient to the fourth decimal place in a pixel.

64 Regarding computed tomography:

A   the cupping effect seen at the centre of a uniform density phantom is caused by hardening of the X-ray beam.

B   quantum mottle is more apparent on a CT image when a wide window width is used.

C   a variation of ±5 Hounsfield units in the water CT number obtained during routine quality control checks is acceptable.

D   a 10% deviation from the expected slice thickness is acceptable during routine quality control checks.

E   the standard deviation of the CT numbers of the pixels in the same region of interest used for water level calibration represents the noise in the image.

65 In computed tomography:

A   statistical noise reduces the contrast resolution of the image.

B   statistical noise is reduced by an increase in pixel size.

C   increasing scanning time reduces statistical noise.

D   reducing slice thickness increases spatial resolution.

E   reducing slice thickness increases contrast resolution.

63 **A** **False** The linear attenuation coefficients of adjacent pixels are independent of each other.

  B **True**

  C **True** The linear attenuation coefficient of a pixel is multiplied by a magnifying constant to give the CT number. Typical CT numbers with a magnification factor of 1000 are: bone (dense)= +1000, intracranial soft tissue = +10 to +50, water = 0, fat = −100, air = −1000.

  D **True**

  E **True**

---

64 **A** **True** As the polyenergetic X-ray beam passes through the uniform density phantom, the lower energy photons are removed and the beam becomes harder with increasing depth. As a result, the pixels near the centre of the image will be assigned smaller values of linear attenuation coefficient than pixels near the periphery. This effect is referred to as cupping.

  B **False** Quantum mottle becomes less apparent when a wide window width is used.

  C **True** This is the maximum limit acceptable. The water CT number calibration is tested by scanning a region of interest of at least several hundred pixels of a circular plastic phantom filled with water.

  D **True** This is the maximum limit acceptable. The slice thickness is assessed by measuring the length of the image of an angulated plate within a special phantom.

  E **True**

---

65 **A** **True**

  B **True** Statistical noise is also reduced by an increase in the slice thickness. Noise is inversely proportional to slice thickness.

  C **True** Increasing the mAs increases the number of photons reaching the detectors and therefore increases the signal to noise ratio.

  D **True**

  E **False** By reducing slice thickness, less emitted quanta are detected and the signal to noise ratio is decreased. This decreases contrast resolution. In addition, reducing slice thickness decreases partial volume effects.

66 Regarding helical CT:

  A it is analogous to spiral CT.

  B it operates at a significantly higher kVp than conventional CT.

  C slip-ring technology is employed in a helical CT scanner to allow the gantry to be rotated continually in a given direction.

  D a full data set of 360° projections is acquired through the same planar section as the reconstructed slice.

  E the pitch of a helical scan is given by the table increment per 360° rotation of the X-ray tube divided by the collimation.

67 The following statements are true regarding diagnostic ultrasound:

  A ultrasound waves are longitudinal waves.

  B the unit of frequency Hertz (Hz) is 10^3 cycles per second.

  C over 99% of the ultrasound beam is reflected at a soft tissue–water interface.

  D in soft tissues the speed of transmission of the ultrasound beam is over 15 000 metres per second.

  E the speed of transmission of the ultrasound beam in soft tissues will increase with increasing frequency of the transducer.

68 Regarding diagnostic ultrasound:

  A a pulsed wave transducer cannot be used to detect the Doppler shift.

  B in a continuous wave transducer two piezoelectric crystals are used.

  C the pulsed wave transducer has a backing which is made of a dense damping material.

  D intensity decays smoothly with distance within the Fresnel zone (near field) of the ultrasonic beam.

  E the limit of axial (depth) resolution for a scanner is approximately half the spatial pulse length.

66 A True
    B False   Helical CT operates at a similar kVp to that used in conventional CT.
    C True   In a slip-ring gantry the electrical connections to the X-ray tube and detector array are achieved using a circular contact with sliding brushes. Due to this arrangement the gantry can be rotated continually in a given direction.
    D False   During helical scanning the patient table is advanced while the gantry is rotated, thus continually acquiring the data in a helical fashion around the patient. To reconstruct planar sections the raw helical data is interpolated so as to approximate the acquisition of a full data set of 360° projections.
    E True   For example, a pitch of 1 means the table increment per 360° rotation of the X-ray tube (measured in mm) is equal to the slice thickness (measured in mm).

67 A True   The disturbance is in the same direction as that of the propagation of the wave.
    B False   1 Hz is 1 cycle per second.
    C False   Less than 1% of the ultrasound beam is reflected at a soft tissue–water interface. Over 99% of the ultrasound beam is reflected at a soft tissue–air interface.
    D False   In the majority of soft tissues the speed of transmission is just over 1500 metres per second.
    E False   The speed of ultrasound in soft tissue is essentially constant and is independent of the frequency used.

68 A False   A continuous wave or pulsed wave ultrasound transducer may be used in modern studies to detect the Doppler shift.
    B True   One crystal is used to transmit the ultrasound beam and the other is used to receive the returning echoes.
    C True
    D False   Intensity decays smoothly with distance in the Frauenhoffer zone (far field) of the ultrasonic beam, which lies beyond the Fresnel zone (near field). The Frauenhoffer zone consists of a divergent main lobe and a number of relatively weak side lobes. Complex intensity variations result from interference effects in the Fresnel zone immediately in front of the transducer.
    E True

69 Regarding the ultrasound transducer:

A the majority of diagnostic ultrasound machines operate at frequencies between 1–10 MHz.

B the bandwidth refers to the complete range of frequencies generated by the transducer.

C the lateral resolution is independent of the beam width.

D the side lobes of the ultrasound beam are occasionally responsible for image artefacts.

E the ultrasound pulse length is kept to a minimum to optimise the axial resolution of the transducer.

70 The following statements are true regarding diagnostic ultrasound:

A for a 2 MHz transducer a 2 cycle pulse lasts for 1×10^{-6} seconds.

B the frequency of the transducer is also known as the pulse repetition frequency (PRF).

C by increasing the PRF from 10 000 to 100 000 pulses per second a significant improvement in the image resolution can be achieved.

D the intensity (or power) of a continuous ultrasound beam is measured in number of pulses per square centimetre.

E for a continuous wave transducer the intensity or power is usually measured close to the transducer surface.

69 **A** **True**
  B **True**
  C **False** The lateral resolution is the resolution across the beam. This resolution depends on the effective beam width at the depth of the target.
  D **True** Image artefacts occur when highly reflective structures fall within the side lobes and return high amplitude echoes to the transducer. These are then registered on the screen and create artefacts.
  E **True** If the pulses are unduly long (i.e. of the order of hundreds of microseconds) the ultrasound equipment will be less able to determine the position of an interface with a high degree of accuracy and thus the axial resolution will be reduced.

70 **A** **True**
  B **False** The frequency with which the pulses are transmitted is termed the pulse repetition frequency (PRF).
  C **False** No significant improvement of the image quality can be achieved beyond a certain PRF value. The general range of PRF is from 500 to 1500 per second.
  D **False** The intensity or power is measured in milliwatts (mW) per square centimetre.
  E **True**

71   Regarding the Doppler effect:

A   the apparent frequency of a signal is altered if the source of the signal is moving with respect to the observer.

B   the frequency of the reflected ultrasound waves decreases if the interface is moving towards the transducer.

C   the magnitude of the increase in the frequency is directly proportional to the velocity of the moving object.

D   the frequency shift depends on the sine of the angle between the ultrasound beam and the direction of movement of the blood when used to measure blood flow.

E   aliasing arises when the Doppler shift frequency exceeds half the pulse repetition frequency (PRF) of the interrogating ultrasound beam.

72   The following statements are true:

A   the angular frequency of precession of a nucleus is determined by the product of the gyromagnetic ratio of the nuclear species and the external field strength.

B   for the field strengths typically used in MR imaging applications, the proton Larmor frequency lies in the range 2–80 MHz.

C   the gyromagnetic ratio of hydrogen (^{1}H) is 42.57 MHz/T.

D ^{1}H has a lower gyromagnetic ratio than those of ^{13}C, ^{15}N, or ^{31}P.

E   the relative atomic abundance of ^{12}C in living tissue is higher than that of ^{1}H.

73   Regarding the angular momentum of the nucleus:

A   it depends on the spin of unpaired protons and neutrons.

B   it depends on the orbital motion of the nucleons (protons and neutrons).

C   the nuclear spin value (I) is always zero or a whole number.

D   it is essential for the precession of the nucleus when placed in a magnetic field.

E   nuclei with a nuclear spin value (I) of zero are suitable for MRI.

71 **A** True
 B False   The reflected frequency increases if the interface is moving towards the transducer and vice versa.
 C True   The shift frequency is also directly proportional to the original ultrasound frequency used.
 D False   It depends on the cosine of the angle between the ultrasound beam and the direction of movement of the blood (beam/vessel angle, θ). Therefore, the maximum Doppler frequency shift is obtained when θ is 0° and so cosine θ is 1. Conversely, when θ is 90°, then cosine θ is 0 and no Doppler signal is obtained. In clinical Doppler examinations, it is important to keep θ as low as possible so as to maximise the Doppler signal.
 E True   There are several approaches to overcome aliasing in clinical practice. The PRF may be increased if the ultrasound equipment permits or the Doppler shift frequency may be reduced. The shift frequency may be reduced by using a lower ultrasound transmission frequency or by increasing the beam/vessel angle (θ).

---

72 **A** True   This is the Larmor equation. Therefore the precessional frequency of a nucleus increases linearly with increasing external magnetic field strength.
 B True
 C True
 D False   The gyromagnetic ratio of ^{13}C is 10.7 MHz/T. The gyromagnetic ratio of ^{15}N is 4.31 MHz/T. The gyromagnetic ratio of ^{31}P is 17.24 MHz/T.
 E False   The relative atomic abundance of ^1H is 1.0 whilst the relative atomic abundance of ^{12}C is 0.19. Of all the most abundant elements in man, ^1H has the most promising nuclear properties for MRI.

---

73 **A** True   This is referred to as the spin angular momentum.
 B True   This is referred to as the orbital angular momentum. It is actually caused by the spinning motion of the entire nucleus rather than by the independent motion of the individual nucleons.
 C False   The nuclear spin value (I) is always zero, a multiple of 1/2 or a whole number.
 D True
 E False   Nuclei with a nuclear spin value of zero do not precess in a magnetic field. Nuclei with spin values of other than zero are suitable for MRI.

74 **When a radiofrequency pulse is applied to a tissue slice within an MR magnet:**

A resonance does not occur if the energy is delivered at a different frequency to that of the Larmor frequency of the nucleus.

B resonance does not occur if the energy is delivered at an angle other than 90° to the net magnetisation vector (NMV).

C during the process of resonance the alignment of the NMV of protons and the external magnetic field is unchanged.

D at a flip angle of 45° the longitudinal NMV is completely transformed into a transverse NMV.

E as a result of resonance the magnetic moments of the nuclei within the transverse NMV move into phase with each other.

75 **Regarding spin echo pulse sequences:**

A the recovery time constant T1 is the time it takes for 50% of the longitudinal magnetisation to recover in the tissue.

B the T1 recovery is also termed the spin–lattice relaxation.

C during free induction decay (FID) the magnitude of the voltage in the receiver coil is reduced as the magnitude of transverse magnetisation decreases.

D the repetition time (TR) of the radiofrequency (RF) pulse has a value of more than 5 seconds.

E the echo time (TE) is the time from application of the RF pulse to the peak of the signal induced in the receiver coil.

76 **In magnetic resonance imaging (MRI):**

A spin–spin relaxation describes the decay of transverse magnetisation.

B the relaxation time constant T2 is the time it takes for 63% of the transverse magnetisation to be lost.

C T1, T2 and T2* rate constants describe exponential decays.

D the time constant T2 is always shorter than the time constant T1 in biological materials.

E the time constant T2* is always longer than the time constant T2 in practice.

74 A True
B True
C False   As a result of resonance the NMV moves out of alignment away from the direction of the external magnetic field.
D False   This only occurs when the flip angle is 90°.
E True

75 A False   It is the time needed for 63% of the longitudinal magnetisation to recover.
B True   The recovery of the longitudinal magnetisation is termed T1 recovery. T1 recovery is caused by the resonant nuclei sharing their excess energy with the surrounding environment or lattice and is termed spin–lattice relaxation.
C True   A signal or voltage is only induced in the receiver coil if the magnetisation in the transverse plane is in phase.
D False   The TR is measured in milliseconds. Typical values: long TR 2000 ms, short TR 250–700 ms.
E True   Typical values: long TE 80 ms; short TE 10–25 ms.

76 A True   Spin–spin relaxation is also termed T2 decay. The decay of transverse magnetisation is caused by the redistribution of excess energy among other resonant nuclei which are relatively less excited.
B True
C True
D True
E False   In practice, the time constant T2* is shorter than the time constant T2. This is because loss of spin coherence is influenced by other factors, such as local magnetic field inhomogeneities, in addition to spin–spin interactions. The time constant T2* denotes the observed decay constant.

77   In a spin echo pulse sequence:

A   hydrogen in water loses transverse magnetisation faster than the hydrogen in fat.

B   the T1 recovery of fat is shorter than the T1 recovery of water.

C   the T2 decay time of water is approximately 5 ms.

D   the T2 decay time of fat is approximately 80 ms.

E   the strength of signal produced in a T1-weighted image is proportional to the amount of transverse magnetisation produced after application of the RF pulse.

78   Regarding parameters affecting the MR image:

A   an increase in the field of view (FOV) decreases the signal to noise ratio.

B   the signal to noise ratio increases as the square of the number of excitations.

C   the signal to noise ratio is reduced in direct proportion to a decrease in slice thickness.

D   the signal to noise ratio increases as the data acquisition bandwidth decreases.

E   an increase in the field of view can be used to overcome an aliasing artefact.

79   Regarding magnetic resonance imaging (MRI):

A   a permanent magnet has the best temporal stability compared with other types of magnet.

B   a resistive magnet is cooled using cryogenic fluids such as liquid helium and liquid nitrogen.

C   iron-cored resistive magnets can operate at field strengths up to 0.5 Tesla.

D   the magnetic field requires a homogeneity of 0.1 parts per million.

E   in vivo spectrometry requires a magnet with a field strength between 0.1 and 0.2 Tesla.

77 A False Hydrogen in fat recovers more rapidly along the longitudinal axis than water and loses transverse magnetisation faster than water.

B True Therefore fat has higher signal on T1-weighted SE sequences than water.

C False The T2 decay time of water is approximately 200 ms.

D True

E True For example, there is more transverse magnetisation in fat than in water after the RF pulse. Fat therefore has a higher signal and appears brighter than water in a T1-weighted image.

78 A False An increase in the FOV increases the voxel volume. Large voxels contain more spins than small voxels and therefore have a higher signal to noise ratio.

B False The signal to noise ratio increases as the square root of the number of excitations. The number of excitations refers to the number of times each value of phase encode is repeated.

C True i.e. thin slice images are noisy.

D True Reducing the data acquisition bandwidth results in less noise being sampled relative to signal. However, chemical shift artefact increases as a consequence.

E True An aliasing artefact occurs because the imaged object is larger than the chosen field of view.

79 A False A superconducting electromagnet has the best temporal stability.

B False A resistive magnet is water cooled while a superconducting electromagnet is cooled using cryogenic fluids.

C True

D False The field homogeneity needed is 10 parts per million.

E False The field strength required is in the region of 1–2 Tesla.

80 In a MRI scanner:

A   the gradient coils, shim coils and radiofrequency coils lie
outside the magnet.

B   there are three sets of gradient coils.

C   a gradient field is used to perform slice selection.

D   slice thickness can be altered by changing the bandwidth of
the applied radiofrequency pulse.

E   shim coils are used to perform frequency encoding and phase
encoding.

81 Regarding a gamma camera detector system:

A   sensitivity and spatial resolution are independent of each other.

B   its resolution is equal to the square root of the sum of the
squares of the intrinsic gamma camera and collimator
resolutions.

C   its spatial resolution increases with an increase in the
collimator-to-object distance.

D   it produces approximately 40 visible light photons for each
incident 140 keV gamma photon that it detects.

E   pulse height analysis is used to select those photomultiplier
tubes (PMTs) in the detector head which have detected a
scintillation.

80 A False   The gradient coils, shim coils and radiofrequency coils must all lie within the inside diameter of the magnet.

   B True   A gradient coil generates a transient change in the magnetic field which varies (approximately) linearly with position along the axis of the magnet bore. It thus produces a field gradient. The three sets of coils generate field gradients in directions perpendicular to each other.

   C True   A gradient field is superimposed on the external magnetic field. Protons along this gradient field are exposed to different magnetic field strengths and therefore have different precession frequencies. A slice can be selectively excited by transmitting a radiofrequency pulse with frequencies corresponding to the precessional frequencies of the protons in that particular slice.

   D True   Slice thickness can also be altered by modifying the steepness of the gradient field.

   E False   Gradient coils are used to perform frequency encoding and phase encoding. Shim coils are used to achieve better magnetic field homogeneity. This process is called shimming.

---

81 A False   High sensitivity is associated with poor spatial resolution and vice versa.

   B True

   C False   Its spatial resolution decreases with an increase in the collimator-to-object distance. This is true for all types of collimator.

   D False   The detector system produces approximately 4000 visible light photons for each incident gamma photon that it detects.

   E False   Pulse height analysis is used to select those pulses generated by the PMTs which correspond to the gamma ray energy of the radionuclide being emitted. In principle, pulse height analysis allows discrimination between scattered and unscattered monoenergetic gamma rays.

82 The scintillation crystal in a gamma camera:
   A has a high density and a high atomic number.
   B is a pure sodium iodide (NaI) crystal.
   C is typically 9–12 mm thick.
   D must be placed in a hermetically sealed container.
   E has an improved sensitivity when it is thick rather than thin.

83 Regarding a gamma camera collimator:
   A a parallel hole collimator forms an image by refracting gamma rays and bringing them into focus at the sodium iodide detector surface.
   B a high resolution collimator has a low sensitivity.
   C a slant hole collimator should be used for gated cardiac acquisitions.
   D a fan beam collimator helps to keep the temperature of the gamma camera electronics low.
   E by increasing the length and number of the collimator holes the intrinsic resolution of the gamma camera can be improved.

84 Regarding Single Photon Emission Computed Tomography (SPECT):
   A a single headed gamma camera must always rotate a full 360° around the patient to register a SPECT acquisition.
   B the most widespread mode of tomographic acquisition is the step-and-shoot method.
   C a multiple headed gamma camera increases the acquisition time as compared with a single headed gamma camera because comparatively more gamma rays will need to be detected.
   D a single headed SPECT camera can only follow a circular or elliptical orbit around the patient.
   E the centre of rotation (COR) correction is stored in the computer memory at the time of installation and is applied to all subsequent SPECT studies.

82 **A** **Irue** This ensures that the crystal has a high stopping efficiency for gamma rays for a given crystal thickness. The high atomic number favours a photoelectric interaction which results in a light pulse that is proportional to the gamma ray energy.

    B **False** The scintillation crystal is a sodium iodide (NaI) crystal doped with approximately 0.1% thallium (TI). The thallium increases the light output from the crystal.

    C **True**

    D **True** The NaI(TI) crystal is hygroscopic.

    E **True** However, a thicker scintillation crystal degrades intrinsic resolution and therefore the crystal thickness that is chosen represents a compromise.

---

83 **A** **False** A parallel hole collimator works on the principle of an absorptive collimation. Unlike visible light, gamma rays cannot be refracted.

    B **True** Increased resolution can only be achieved by reducing the overall sensitivity.

    C **True** A 15° slant hole collimator is best suited for separating the left atrium from the left ventricle.

    D **False** A fan beam collimator refers to the arrangement of individual collimator septa and is used for cardiac and cerebral SPECT imaging. Collimators do not control the temperature of the electronics.

    E **False** The intrinsic resolution of the gamma camera is a function of the sodium iodide crystal thickness, number and shape of the photomultiplier tubes and associated electronics. The collimator characteristics do not affect intrinsic resolution.

---

84 **A** **False** A SPECT acquisition can be performed by a gamma camera rotating 180° around the patient (e.g. myocardial perfusion study: 180° rotation).

    B **True**

    C **False** A multiple headed gamma camera is much faster than a single headed camera because multiple projections can be acquired simultaneously.

    D **False** Modern SPECT camera heads can follow an operator defined contour around the patient. This reduces the distance between the detector and the gamma camera thus preventing loss of resolution.

    E **False** The extent of COR correction can change with time. Therefore the COR correction is assessed on a regular basis (e.g. at least once a week) and then stored on the computer. It is applied to the SPECT images during the reconstruction process.

85   Regarding positron emission tomography (PET):

A   a positron has a unit positive charge and no mass.

B   a neutron is converted into a positron and a proton during positron emission.

C   the scintillation detector is usually made of bismuth germanate.

D   the positron decay is detected by a coincident detection method.

E   the positron emitters that are used in PET imaging have longer half-lives than that of ^{99m}Tc.

86   Regarding the handling of unsealed radionuclides:

A   the administered activity is measured using a scintillation detector.

B   the performance of an isotope calibrator is independent of the source geometry.

C   mouth pipetting of radioactive liquids with low specific activities is permissible provided that it is performed in a well ventilated fume cupboard.

D   lead syringe shields are used during the dispensing of radiopharmaceuticals.

E   routine contamination monitoring of controlled areas is performed using a calibrated dose rate meter.

87   Regarding patient dose resulting from the administration of a radiopharmaceutical:

A   the dose received depends on the decay scheme of the radionuclide.

B   the absorbed dose is directly proportional to the amount of radioactivity administered.

C   the patient dose can be decreased by reducing the acquisition times using a gamma camera.

D   for ARSAC recommended doses the effective dose equivalent (EDE) is always less than 5 mSv.

E   the biological half-life does not affect the absorbed dose.

85 **A** **False**   A positron has a unit positive charge and the same mass as that of an electron.

  B **False**   During positron emission a proton is converted into a neutron and a positron. A positron and a neutrino are ejected from the nucleus.

  C **True**   The high atomic number of bismuth (Z = 83) and the high density of the crystal give a high intrinsic detection efficiency for 511 keV photons. These photons are produced by the positron annihilation process.

  D **True**

  E **False**   The radionuclides used in PET imaging have very short half-lives, e.g. ^{11}C (20.5 min), ^{13}N (10 min), ^{15}O (2 min), ^{18}F (110 min). The half-life of ^{99m}Tc is 6 hours.

---

86 **A** **False**   Activity is measured using a calibrated isotope calibrator.

  B **False**   Isotope calibrator performance depends on the source geometry. Different calibration factors are used for the same radionuclide presented in different geometries, i.e. ^{99m}Tc activities measured in a syringe and in a vial require the use of different calibration factors.

  C **False**   Mouth pipetting of radioactive liquids is not permitted under any circumstances.

  D **True**   The use of lead or tungsten syringe shields reduces finger dose.

  E **False**   A calibrated contamination monitor (not a dose rate meter) for appropriate radionuclides is used.

---

87 **A** **True**   The type of radiation emitted and the presence of radioactive daughter products will influence the absorbed radiation dose.

  B **True**

  C **False**   Patient dose is independent of the image acquisition times using a gamma camera. It depends primarily on the amount of radiopharmaceutical administered and other measures taken to reduce patient dose (e.g. thyroid blocking agents).

  D **False**   For example, the dose due to ^{201}Tl used in myocardial imaging is higher, i.e. 20mSv.

  E **False**   A shorter biological half-life reduces the absorbed dose.

88   Regarding radiation doses:

A   the average total annual radiation dose to a member of the UK population is 2.5 mSv.

B   nuclear fall out and discharges account for the largest man-made contribution to the radiation burden of the population living in developed countries.

C   the average effective dose from a skull radiograph is approximately 0.15 mSv.

D   the average effective dose from an IVU examination is approximately 3.5 mSv.

E   the average effective dose from a ^{99m}Tc MDP bone scan is approximately 15 mSv.

89   The effective dose:

A   is the same as the effective dose equivalent.

B   of an abdominal radiograph is approximately 1.5 mSv.

C   of a barium enema is equivalent to approximately 4.5 years natural background radiation.

D   of a chest CT scan is equivalent to approximately 40 PA chest films.

E   of a ^{201}Tl myocardial perfusion scan is less than that of a ^{99m}Tc methoxy isobutyl isonitrile (MIBI) myocardial perfusion scan.

90   Regarding the radiation monitoring film badge:

A   the X-ray film used inside the badge has a fast emulsion on one side and a slow emulsion on the other side.

B   the cadmium-lead filter is used to estimate the exposure to thermal neutrons.

C   the photographic film becomes progressively less optically dense as a result of exposure to ionising radiations.

D   the use of plastic, tin and aluminium filters in a film badge enables the distinction to be made between X-ray and ultraviolet exposures.

E   the film badges are calibrated by exposing some badges from the batch to a known amount of radiation.

88 A **True**
    B **False**   Medical irradiation contributes up to 90% of the total
                    man-made radiation dose.
    C **True**   The effective dose is a measure of the combined
                    effect on the whole body of the radiation doses to
                    several different organs or tissues in the body.
    D **True**
    E **False**   The effective dose from a ^{99m}Tc MDP bone scan is
                    approximately 5 mSv.

89 A **True**   The 1990 Recommendations of the International
                    Commission on Radiological Protection (ICRP
                    Publication 60) now use the term effective dose,
                    which is analogous to the term effective dose
                    equivalent used in previous ICRP publications.
    B **True**
    C **True**   The effective dose of a barium enema is
                    approximately 9 mSv.
    D **False**   The effective doses of a chest CT and a PA chest film
                    are approximately 8 mSv and 0.02 mSv respectively.
                    Therefore the dose of one chest CT is equivalent to
                    that of 400 chest films.
    E **False**   The effective dose of a ^{201}Tl myocardial perfusion
                    scan is approximately 20 mSv. The effective dose of
                    a ^{99m}Tc MIBI myocardial perfusion scan is
                    approximately 4 mSv.

90 A **True**   If a high exposure of radiation has occurred, the fast
                    emulsion can be removed and an estimate of the
                    dose can then be made from the measurements on
                    the slow emulsion.
    B **True**   The neutron capture by cadmium nuclei results in
                    gamma emission which exposes the film.
    C **False**   The photographic film becomes progressively more
                    dense as a result of exposure to ionising radiations.
    D **False**   The different filters allow the distinction to be made
                    as to whether the dose was the result of beta particle
                    emission, high or low energy X-rays, or gamma rays.
    E **True**

91   An air equivalent wall ionisation chamber:

A   is unsuitable for measurement of radiation at the higher kilovoltages used in diagnostic radiology.

B   is more sensitive than a Geiger counter.

C   can be used to measure exposure rates.

D   may be converted into a chamber whose response varies with photon energy in the same way as the standard air chamber.

E   requires high gas pressure inside the chamber.

92   Regarding radiation protection:

A   the radiation weighting factors (quality factors) depend on the relative biological effectiveness (RBE) of the radiation.

B   the radiation weighting factor (quality factor) for X-rays is 0.5.

C   the annual whole body dose limit for a member of the public is ten times less than that for a radiation worker.

D   the average annual whole body dose per person in the UK due to natural background radiation is 10 mSv.

E   exposure to natural background radiation mainly arises from ^{222}Rn, ^{40}K and ^{14}C.

93   The radiation weighting factor (quality factor) is:

A   dependent on the relative biological effectiveness.

B   greater for radiations with a low linear energy transfer.

C   a factor determining equivalent dose.

D   higher for all particulate radiations than it is for ^{60}Co gamma emission.

E   considered to be constant for the diagnostic range of X-rays.

91 **A** **False** An ionisation chamber is suitable for measurement of radiation at all kilovoltages used in diagnostic radiology.

  B **False** The amount of an electrical charge or current released in an ionisation chamber is very small. Unlike the Geiger counter, the ionisation chamber cannot be used to count individual radiation events. Instead the total amount of current passing through the chamber can be measured using an electrometer.

  C **True**

  D **True** By adjusting the size of the aluminium electrode and the amount of carbon.

  E **False** The gas used is air at atmospheric pressure.

---

92 **A** **True** The RBE of the radiation is a ratio of the dose from standard radiation (usually 200 kVp X-rays) to produce a given biological effect to the dose from the test radiation to produce the same biological effect.

  B **False** The radiation weighting factor for X-rays (and gamma rays and beta particles) is 1.

  C **True** The annual whole body dose limit for a radiation worker is 50 mSv. The annual whole body dose limit for a member of the public is 5 mSv (Ionising Radiations Regulations 1985).

  D **False** The UK population average annual whole body dose due to the natural background radiation is approximately 2.175 mSv.

  E **True**

---

93 **A** **True**

  B **False** It is greater for radiations with higher linear energy transfer.

  C **True**

  D **False** The quality factor for electrons (except Auger electrons emitted from nuclei bound to DNA) is the same as that for ^{60}Co gamma emissions.

  E **True**

94   Radiation dose to the patient in diagnostic radiography can be reduced by:
  A   reducing scatter with a grid.
  B   decreasing the object to film distance.
  C   compressing the abdomen during an IVU examination.
  D   using rare-earth phosphors in the screen.
  E   selecting the highest tube voltage consistent with acceptable image quality.

95   Regarding diagnostic imaging:
  A   thermionic emission is preceded by electronic excitation.
  B   a large proportion of the energy in the incident X-ray beam is converted to heat energy in the tissues.
  C   gamma emissions from ^{99m}Tc have a higher linear energy transfer (LET) than 100 kVp X-rays.
  D   small temperature changes in irradiated gonads are thought to be responsible for the consequent genetic effects.
  E   dehydrated patients are at a higher risk of radiation-induced damage.

96   Regarding the biological effects of radiation:
  A   the severity of stochastic effects is dose dependent.
  B   Cancer induction is an example of a non-stochastic effect.
  C   All the somatic effects of radiation are stochastic.
  D   radiation dose levels in diagnostic radiology are more likely to produce non-stochastic effects than stochastic effects.
  E   gamma emissions from radionuclide imaging are more likely to produce non-stochastic effects than are X-rays.

97   The following statements are true of the non-stochastic effects of radiation:
  A   there is a threshold dose below which non-stochastic effects do not occur.
  B   the severity of the effects is at least in part dose dependent.
  C   the effects are assumed to be non-additive if the time interval between the exposures is sufficiently long to permit complete recovery.
  D   a pleural effusion following radiotherapy is an example of a non-stochastic effect.
  E   skin erythema is an example of a non-stochastic effect.

94 **A** **False** A grid always absorbs some primary radiation in addition to scattered radiation and therefore exposure factors need to be increased when a grid is used. This increases the radiation dose to the patient.

    B **True**

    C **True**

    D **True**

    E **True**

95 **A** **True**

    B **True**

    C **False** The LET is the number of keV lost per micron of track of ionising radiation. It is similar for X-rays and gamma rays.

    D **False** Temperature changes are insignificant. Genetic damage is caused by the interactions between ionising radiation and the genetic material of the germ cells.

    E **False** The state of hydration is not relevant.

96 **A** **False** The severity of stochastic effects is not dose dependent. The probability of the effect occurring is dose dependent without a threshold.

    B **False** Cancer induction in somatic tissue is a stochastic effect of radiation. Genetic effects are also stochastic.

    C **False** The somatic effects of radiation are both stochastic and non-stochastic.

    D **False** The reverse is true.

    E **False** Gamma emissions and X-rays are both equally likely to produce non-stochastic effects.

97 **A** **True** Above the threshold dose, non-stochastic effects occur with a high degree of predictability.

    B **True** When the threshold dose level is exceeded, the severity of the non-stochastic effects is proportional to the radiation dose.

    C **True**

    D **True**

    E **True** Cataract formation is another example of a non-stochastic effect of radiation.

98   Regarding radiation protection legislation:

   A   the POPUMET regulations (1988) are concerned with the radiation protection of radiation workers.

   B   the Radioactive Substances Act (1993) does not apply to hospitals.

   C   the ARSAC issues licences to administer radioactive substances under the Medicines Act (1978).

   D   the Radioactive Material (Road Transport) Act (1991) only applies to the nuclear power industry.

   E   the Ionising Radiations Regulations (1985) are designed to protect the public as well as staff.

99   Regarding the statutory radiation dose limits (IRR 1985):

   A   for radiation workers the dose limit for the lens of the eye is 15 mSv per year.

   B   the whole body annual dose limit for a trainee radiation worker aged under 18 years is the same as that for a radiation worker aged 30 years.

   C   the dose limit for the abdomen of a pregnant woman is 10 mSv during the declared term of pregnancy.

   D   the whole body dose limit for a classified worker is 5 mSv per year.

   E   a radiation dose below these statutory limits is considered to be free of any harm.

100   Regarding the Ionising Radiation (POPUMET) Regulations 1988:

   A   medically qualified persons can direct medical exposure for a diagnostic purpose without any additional training.

   B   they do not apply to the in vitro use of ionising radiation in scientific research.

   C   it is the duty of the employer to maintain an up to date inventory of the X-ray equipment.

   D   the core of knowledge training records of all staff who are involved in clinically or physically directing radiation dose are maintained by the employer.

   E   responsibility for medical exposure lies solely with the person physically directing it.

98 A **False** The POPUMET regulations (1988) are concerned with the protection of persons undergoing medical examination or treatment.
    B **False** The Radioactive Substances Act (1993) applies to all work places involved in the use of radioactive substances.
    C **True**
    D **False** The act equally applies to hospitals which transport radioactive materials. Note that the Radioactive Material (Road Transport)(Great Britain) Regulations became law in 1995.
    E **True**

99 A **False** The limit is set at 150 mSv per year.
    B **False** The whole body dose limit for a trainee radiation worker aged under 18 years is 15 mSv per year; this is less than the limit for a radiation worker aged over 18 years (50 mSv per year).
    C **True** Note also that the dose limit to the abdomen of women of reproductive capacity is set at 13 mSv in any three consecutive months.
    D **False** The whole body dose limit for a classified worker is 50 mSv per year.
    E **False** No level of radiation dose is considered to be safe for stochastic effects.

100 A **False** According to the POPUMET Regulations 1988 all persons directing clinical or physical exposure need to be adequately trained to acquire a core of knowledge in radiation protection matters.
    B **True**
    C **True**
    D **True**
    E **False** The responsibility lies with the person clinically directing it. The person physically directing it is required to keep the dose as low as reasonably practicable.

Bibliography

Administration of Radioactive Substances Advisory Committee (ARSAC). Notes for Guidance on the Administration of Radioactive Substances to Persons for Purposes of Diagnosis, Treatment or Research. London: Department of Health, 1993.

Agur AMR. Grant's Atlas of Anatomy. 9th edn. Baltimore: Williams and Wilkins, 1991.

Ansell G, Wilkins RA. Complications in Diagnostic Imaging. 2nd edn. Oxford: Blackwell Scientific Publications, 1987.

British Institute of Radiology. Assurance of Quality in the Diagnostic X-ray Department. London: BIR, 1988.

British National Formulary Number 27 (March 1994). London: British Medical Association and the Royal Pharmaceutical Society of Great Britain, 1994.

Bushberg J, Seibert J, Leidholdt E, Boone J. The Essential Physics of Medical Imaging. Baltimore: Williams and Wilkins, 1994.

Caffey J. Paediatric X-ray Diagnosis. 8th edn. Chicago: Year Book Medical Publishers, 1985.

Chapman S, Nakielny R. A Guide to Radiological Procedures. 3rd edn. London: Baillière Tindall, 1993.

Chesney D, Chesney M. Radiographic Imaging. 4th edn. Oxford: Blackwell Scientific Publications, 1981.

Clark KC. Positioning in Radiography. 9th edn. London: William Heinemann Medical Books, 1974.

Cosgrove D, Meire H, Dewbury K. Clinical Ultrasound: Abdominal and General Ultrasound. Edinburgh: Churchill Livingstone, 1992.

Curry TS, Dowdey JE, Murry RC. Christensen's Introduction to the Physics of Diagnostic Radiology. 3rd edn. Philadelphia: Lea and Febiger, 1984.

Dendy PP, Heaton B. Physics for Radiologists. Oxford: Blackwell Scientific Publications, 1987.

Grainger RG, Allison DJ. Diagnostic Radiology. 2nd edn. Edinburgh: Churchill Livingstone, 1992.

Hornsby VPL, Winter RK. Aids to Part I FRCR. Edinburgh: Churchill Livingstone, 1988.

Hospital Physicist's Association. The Physics of Radiodiagnosis. 2nd edn. London: HPA, 1977.

Institute of Physical Sciences in Medicine. Report No. 59. The Commissioning and Routine Testing of Mammographic X-ray Systems. 2nd edn. York: IPSM, 1994.

Institute of Physical Sciences in Medicine. Report No. 67 Quality Assurance in Dental Radiology. York: IPSM, 1994.

Johns H, Cunningham J. The Physics of Radiology. 4th edn. Springfield, Illinois: Charles C. Thomas, 1983.

Keats TE. Atlas of Normal Roentgen Variants That May Simulate Disease. 4th edn. Chicago: Year Book Medical Publications, 1988.

Maisey M, Britton K, Gllady D. Clinical Nuclear Medicine. 2nd edn. London: Chapman and Hall, 1991.

Martin A, Harbison S. An Introduction to Radiation Protection. 3rd edn. London: Chapman and Hall, 1986.

McMinn RMH. Last's Anatomy. 8th edn. Edinburgh: Churchill Livingstone, 1990.

Meschan I. An Atlas of Normal Radiographic Anatomy. 2nd edn. London: W B Saunders, 1959.

Moores B, Henshaw E, Watkinson S, Pearcy B. Practical Guide to Quality Assurance in Medical Imaging. Chichester: John Wiley and Sons, 1987.

Moores B, Stieve F, Eriskat H, Schibilla H. The BIR Report 18. Technical and Physical Parameters in Medical Diagnostic Radiology. London: BIR, 1989.

RCR Working Party. Making the Best Use of a Department of Clinical Radiology: Guidelines for Doctors. 3rd edn. London: Royal College of Radiologists, 1995.

Sander RC. Clinical Sonography: A Practical Guide. 2nd edn. Boston: Little, Brown and Company, 1991.

Sharp PF, Gemmell HG, Smith FW. Practical Nuclear Medicine. Oxford: IRL Press, 1989.

Sorenson J, Phelps M. Physics in Nuclear Medicine. New York: Grune and Stratton, 1980.

The Ionising Radiation (Protection of Persons Undergoing Medical Examination or Treatment) Regulations. Statutory Instrument No. 778. London: HMSO, 1988.

The Ionising Radiations Regulations. Statutory Instrument No. 1333. London: HMSO, 1985.

Webb S. The Physics of Medical Imaging. Bristol: Adam Hilger, 1988.

Weir J, Abrahams PH. An Imaging Atlas of Human Anatomy. London: Wolfe, 1992.

Westacott S, Hall JRW. Key Anatomy for Radiology. Oxford: Heinemann Medical Books, 1988.

Westbrook C, Kaut C. MRI in Practice. Oxford: Blackwell Scientific Publications, 1993.

Whitehouse GH, Worthington BS. Techniques in Diagnostic Imaging. 2nd edn. Oxford: Blackwell Scientific Publications, 1990.

Wilks R. Principles of Radiological Physics. 2nd edn. Edinburgh: Churchill Livingstone, 1987.

Wotton R. Radiation Protection of Patients. Cambridge: Cambridge University Press, 1993.

The FRCR part I syllabus

The Royal College of Radiologists has kindly given permission to the authors to include the present FRCR part I syllabus in this book. It should be noted that this book is not an official publication of the Royal College of Radiologists, and detailed information on any aspect of the fellowship examination and the syllabus should be obtained from:

> The Examinations Secretary,
> The Royal College of Radiologists,
> 38, Portland Place,
> London W1N 4JQ.

1.0 RADIOLOGICAL ANATOMY AND TECHNIQUES

1.1 Radiological anatomy

General comments
The candidate should be familiar not only with the basic anatomy relevant to all the common radiological examinations but should also be familiar with cross-sectional anatomy in the axial, coronal, sagittal and, where appropriate, oblique planes. A knowledge of normal anatomical variations will be expected. It is expected that the formal teaching course will build on the anatomical knowledge already expected of a radiological trainee, in much the same way as the interpretation of radiological abnormalities is built on a sound knowledge of basic pathology.

Candidates should know the normal appearances in the growing child including epiphyseal ossification, but need not memorise the dates of appearance of the ossification centres.

1.1.1 The syllabus for anatomy as shown by imaging examinations includes the following systems:

- The skull including the facial bones, mandible, teeth, lacrimal apparatus
- The remainder of the skeletal system
- The respiratory system
- The abdomen
- The gastro-intestinal tract and biliary system
- The urinary tract
- The cardiovascular system
- The lymphatic system
- The female pelvic organs, including the pregnant uterus
- The anatomy and ultrasound dating of the normal foetus
- The female breast

- The male genital tract
- The brain, spinal cord and meninges
- The endocrine system.

1.2 Radiological techniques

1.2.1 The candidate will be expected to show familiarity with, and experience of, everyday investigations. A detailed knowledge is only required for those techniques which a candidate is expected to have carried out personally and on his/her own during the first 9 months of training in radiology. These examinations are standard contrast examinations of the gastro-intestinal tract, intravenous urography, urethrography, cystography, leg venography, sialography, dacrocystography, hysterosalpingography, T-tube cholangiography, sinography and a nephrostogram.

1.2.2 A knowledge of the basic principles underlying the techniques used in arteriography, interventional radiology, biliary tract imaging, nuclear medicine, ultrasound, CT and MRI will also be expected but in less detail. For these investigations, the candidate should know, in outline only, the following:

- The principal indications and contra-indications
- Patient preparation
- Radiographic apparatus used
- Contrast media (see 1.3 below)
- Outline of technique with main variations
- Principal complications and their treatment.

1.3 Contrast media, radiopharmaceuticals and drugs

1.3.1 Contrast media: The contrast media to be studied are those which relate to the practical procedures mentioned in 1.2 above. They include the contrast media in current clinical use for radiography, computed tomography and magnetic resonance imaging. For each contrast agent the following are expected:

- Official name
- Doses, including doses for children
- Constitution (not the detailed formula)
- Modes of administration and the clinical uses
- Routes of elimination
- Relative advantages of the different types of media
- Side effects and treatment of reactions
- Contra-indications to use.

1.3.2 Radiopharmaceuticals: The choice of radiopharmaceuticals.

1.3.3 Drugs: Some knowledge is expected of those drugs commonly used in radiological practice, including their dosage. These can be considered under the following headings:

- Preparation of the gastro-intestinal tract, including drugs modifying bowel behaviour
- Sedation before radiological procedures
- Prophylaxis and treatment of reactions to contrast media
- Prophylaxis and treatment of reactions to radiological procedures other than to contrast, e.g. in phaeochromocytoma.

1.4 Radiography

General comments
Candidates will be expected to demonstrate a knowledge of the standard radiographic projections relating to the regions outlined in the radiological anatomy syllabus (section 1.1 above). Candidates should, therefore, be able to comment on the positioning and tube angulation used to obtain the image and should be able to give practical advice on improving the quality of the film. A knowledge of infrequently used projections will not be expected.

1.4.1 Knowledge of, and practical familiarity with, the following will be expected:

- Positioning of patients. The use of immobilising devices and protective devices
- Standard radiographic projections and angles. Correction of errors in centering an exposure
- The specific problems of mobile radiographic techniques
- The following standard radiographic projections:
  Basic skull views including the facial bones
  AP and lateral projections of the spine
  PA and lateral chest radiograph
  Erect and supine abdomen
  AP pelvis
  Standard views of the shoulder girdle, pelvic girdle and extremities.

2.0 PHYSICS

General comments

- A basic knowledge of physics is assumed.

- On the assumption that the whole of the physics syllabus can be covered in approximately 40 hours of formal teaching, the hours indicated in brackets are a guide as to how these 40 hours might be divided. The suggested time for each section is an indication of the approximate proportion of questions devoted to each topic in the MCQ part of the examination and the depth of knowledge expected in the topic.

- The changes in content and recommended time contained in this revision of the syllabus are designed to reflect the introduction of the newer imaging modalities.

- Equipment design and construction details will **not** be examined, but an understanding of the **function** of equipment components relevant to image formation may be tested.

- A mathematical approach to the physics syllabus is inappropriate; the emphasis should be placed on a clear understanding of the physical basis of radiological practice in a qualitative sense. However, the knowledge of the approximate magnitude of quantities encountered in daily practice will be expected, e.g. percentage transmission of X-radiation through a patient; the activity of a radionuclide used for bone scanning.

- Basic electricity, magnetism and mathematics are not included in the syllabus and questions on these subjects will not be included in the examination.

- During formal teaching, all physics demonstrations/practicals should have a direct relevance to everyday radiology.

- *Knowledge of the principles of quality assurance, contrast resolution, spatial resolution and noise is expected for all the sections listed below.*

2.1 Ionising radiation (5 hours)

- Structure of the atom.

- Radioactivity and radionuclides: basic definition of alpha, beta and gamma radiation; principles of exponential decay, half-life, specific activity and units of activity.

- Electromagnetic spectrum.

- General properties of X- and gamma rays: wavelength, energy, inverse square law.

- Interaction of X- and gamma rays with matter: coherent, Compton and photoelectric interactions; concepts of attenuation, absorption and scatter — and their practical consequences.

2.2 Radiation protection (7 hours)

- Statutory responsibilities: an appreciation of relevant legislation and Codes of Practice.

- The content of the "core of knowledge" as specified by the Ionising Radiation (POPUMET) Regulations (1988) or subsequent revisions.

- Genetic and somatic effects of ionising radiations.
- Relative risks of ionising radiations.
- The principles of dose limitation, including the various practical means of dose reduction to staff and patient with special consideration of females and children.
- Staff and patient doses: magnitude and measurement.

2.3 Production of X-rays (3 hours)
- The basic principles of a rotating anode X-ray tube.
- Basic factors which influence X-ray output from differing types of X-ray machinery: anode material, kV, mA, focal spot size, tube rating, filtration. (Design and construction details will not be examined.)

2.4 The X-ray image (10 hours)
- Geometric factors and magnification, effect of focal spot size, geometric movement and unsharpness.
- Conventional film/screen systems: basic structure; characteristic curve; latitude; density; speed; contrast and how to influence or manipulate it.
- Basic principles and effects of film processing.
- Basic principles of image intensification. Operator-controlled variables.
- Principles of tomography, particularly CT, with emphasis on operator-controlled variables, e.g. slice thickness, partial volume effect, field size and effect on resolution, data storage and display, pixel/voxel, window width and level, and grey scale.
- Basic principles of digital imaging and picture archiving and communications systems (PACS).

2.5 Principles of diagnostic ultrasound (5 hours)
- The basic components of an ultrasound system.
- Types of transducer and the production of ultrasound with emphasis on operator-controlled variables.
- The frequencies of medical ultrasound.
- The interaction of ultrasound with tissue, including biological effects.
- The basic principles of A, B, M, real-time and duplex scanning.
- The basic principles of pulsed, continuous wave and colour Doppler ultrasound.
- Recognition and explanation of common artefacts.

2.6 Magnetic resonance imaging (5 hours)

- Basic principles and origin of the signal.
- Principles of basic sequences in clinical use.
- Concept of T_1, T_2, proton density and effect of motion on signal.
- Magnetic field hazards to patients, staff and passers by.

2.7 Radionuclide imaging (5 hours)

- The function of a gamma camera.
- Properties of radiopharmaceuticals.
- Static and dynamic imaging.
- Handling of radionuclides.
- Introduction to single photon emission computed tomography (SPECT) and positron emission tomography (PET).

Index

Superior mesenteric artery, 28–9,
32–3
Superior mesenteric vein, 37
Superior vena cava, 16–17, 22–3
filling defects, 128–9
Superior vena cavography, 100–1
Surgical clips, 132–3
Sutural sclerosis, 48–9
Symphysis pubis, 40–1
Syringe shields, lead/tungsten, 196–7
Systemic lupus erythematosus,
intravenous urography, 84–5

Taeniae coli, 28–9
99mTc
DMSA urinary tract examination,
112–13
DTPA, 108–9
aerosol, 110–11
urinary tract examination, 112–13
gamma emissions, 202–3
HMPAO, 108–9
MAG-3 urinary tract examination,
112–13
methoxy isobutyl isonitrile scan,
114–15
methylene diphosphonate, 108–9
MIBI myocardial perfusion scan,
198–9
pertechnetate, 108–9, 110–11, 115
red cell labelling, 115
pyrophosphate, 114–15
sulphur colloid, 114–15
tin colloid, 116–17
99mTc-macroaggregated albumin
particles, 112–13
Teeth, 60–1
occlusal plane, 96–7
Temporomandibular joint, 58–9
articular disc, 58–9
Tendon MRI, 134–5
Terbium ion, 158–9
Testes, 40–1, 44–5
lymphatic drainage, 46–7
ultrasound scanning, 118–19
Thoracic artery, lateral, 22–3
Thoracic duct, 12–13, 14–15, 16–17
Thorax, computed tomography,
124–5, 126–7, 198–9
Thrombus, Doppler imaging of veins,
124–5
Thymus, 18–19
Thyratron, 148–9
Thyrocervical trunk, 18–19

Thyroid, 20–1
angle of laminae, 20–1
cartilage, 20–1
inferior artery, 52–3
isotope examination, 110–11
isthmus, 12–13
ultrasound scanning, 120–1
veins, 20–1
Thyroidea ima artery, 20–1
Tibial vein, anterior, 98–9
Time of flight magnetic resonance
angiography, 134–5
201Tl
image, 110–11
myocardial perfusion scan, 198–9
uptake, 114–15
Tomography, 78–9
Toxic megacolon, 74–5
Trachea, 10–11, 12–13
Tracheo-oesophageal fistula, 66–7,
76–7
Transfemoral puncture, 106–7
Transmission ratio, 152–3
Transrectal guided biopsy, 122–3
Transverse sinus, 22–3
Tri-radiate cartilage, 120–1
Tricuspid valve, 23
Tricyclic antidepressants, 116–17
Triquetrum, 2–3
Triticeal cartilage, 20
Tunica vaginalis, 44–5

Ultrasound
7.5 MHz frequency transducer,
120–1
antenatal, 44–5
axial resolution limit, 182–3
beam
Frauenhoffer zone, 182
Fresnel zone, 182
intensity, 184–5
reflection, 182–3
side lobes, 184–5
transmission speed, 182–3
diagnostic, 182–3, 184–5, 212
Doppler effect, 186–7
endoscopic of oesophagus, 122–3
interventional techniques, 122–3
neonates, 120–1
pancreas, 118–19
pulse
duration, 184–5
length, 184–5
repetition frequency, 184–5